RE

"*Dream, Redefined* feels like a warm hug from Oprah. Sparkling with candor, resiliency, and audacious truth-telling, Candace Clark Trinchieri shares her extraordinary journey in becoming a mom. Interweaving personal narrative with vibrant life stories from other women of color, this book is a powerful testament for all women, reminding us that we are never alone and we are always enough. I freaking love this book!"

-Ellie Knaus | *Atomic Moms* podcast

"A bold, insightful, and illuminating look into navigating infertility as a woman of color. Candace Clark Trinchieri brilliantly weaves together her journey and the experiences of minority women who've been faced with fertility struggles, undergone reproductive technologies, and grieved pregnancy losses. In a book you won't soon forget, she delivers a powerful and much-needed voice for those whose stories are often overlooked. This game-changing book will simultaneously make you laugh out loud and shed tears of resonance, as you revel in narratives that deeply connect to your own experience or those you love. A must read."

-Jessica Zucker, Ph.D. | Author of *I Had a Miscarriage: A Memoir, a Movement*

"For generations, women of color have gone through life dealing with pain and suffering alone and nowhere to tell their stories authentically. Society has attempted to silence those stories for far too long. Just as my podcast provides a safe space for truthful storytelling, *Dream, Redefined* dares to bring change."
-Monique Farook | *Infertility and Me* podcast

"*Dream, Redefined* highlights voices of women of color, yet this is a book for all women struggling with infertility. The bold, vulnerable stories generously shared here would have made my isolating experience (filled with years of shame and pain) a bit more bearable as I navigated through loss after loss, and challenge after challenge. In short, it's the book for which I had been searching and never found."
-Jessica Weinstock | The B(e)ARING All Project

Dream
REDEFINED

THE STRUGGLE AND SUCCESS THROUGH INFERTILITY AS A WOMAN OF COLOR

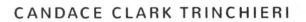

CANDACE CLARK TRINCHIERI

CONTENTS

♥ ♡ ♥ ♡ ♥ ♡ ♥ ♡ ♥

For my parents,
who despite all evidence to the contrary, believe
that I am the perfect daughter.

For Tommaso,
who never let me stop believing.

For Max,
who makes my life beautiful every day in every way.

For all the sons and daughters lost before I had the
chance to kiss them goodnight.

Prologue

BEFORE WE BEGIN

"Everything might not be OKAY for you right now and that's OKAY."

-Unknown

Infertility is tough. Anyone who says otherwise is probably trying to sell you something and it's most likely an overpriced "miracle cure". Absolutely nothing about infertility is easy or fair. I was thirty-eight, newly married, and finally at a point in my life when I was ready to start my family. Everything had fallen into place and having a child was going to be the cherry on top of the pie of my life. So, how did everything that felt so right go so wrong, so quickly? Finding out I was infertile threw me into a tornado that spun my life out of my control. When the storm spat me out, I had a child, but my body and spirit were bruised and bore the scars of two major surgeries, nine In Vitro Fertilization (IVF) attempts, an egg donor, a failed attempt at surrogacy, countless miscarriages, and the mountain of red-tape and paperwork required for adoption. Having a baby was not as easy as they warned me it was going to be in high school. Nothing—absolutely nothing—seemed or felt natural in the pursuit of making a baby.

I won't pretend that I am an expert on everything about infertility; I don't have all the answers. This isn't going to be a medical book or journal, full of facts, figures, or statistics. This is not a book about the "how's" and "why's" of infertility; it won't neatly wrap up with a bow about how to get pregnant and have a child. This is a book about women. Specifically, it's about women of color—their experience, perspective, struggle, and, most importantly, their success in finding peace no matter where their journeys ended up. Like most of us, I am only an expert in my experience. The moment I discovered I was infertile, I wasn't just sad, I was angry. I was so pissed off that my body didn't work the way it was supposed to work and it felt like I had no one to point the finger at but myself. I will be honest: it was pure, unfiltered anger that drove me into all my advocacy efforts. I became involved with RESOLVE, The National Infertility Association, first as an Ambassador and Co-Chair of the Southern California Walk of Hope. I contributed to training hundreds of volunteer advocates for the annual RESOLVE Advocacy Day in Washington, DC as the National Vice-Chair of Policy and Education. I spoke to congressional and Senate leadership about expanding infertility coverage and the Adoption Tax Credit. Back home in Los Angeles, I co-hosted the Infertility Warriors monthly support group (open to all, but geared to women of color) with the amazing Tomiko Frasier Hines. I did all this while actively going through IVF. I remember being stopped at airport security on a trip to advocate in Washington, DC: the estrogen patches strapped around my stomach and waist looked "bomb-like" to security. I may also be one of the few people who has shot up fertility meds in the bathroom of a US Senate building between meeting with Senate and congressional staffers, but I can't be certain. I was a bat out of hell for those first few years and it was the anger that fueled me. Now, I think that a lot of the anger wasn't just for myself—it was also because I never wanted any other woman to go through what I did.

It can be a supreme challenge to move through the world as a woman of color and want to openly share your experiences and see your stories reflected in the world around you. Yet, so often the world seems not quite ready or prepared to hear it. We have all grown so comfortable with certain myths that the reality seems almost impossible to believe. One in eight women experience infertility[1]—that is a well-known truth. Black women are almost twice as likely to be infertile as white women[2]—that is a little-known fact. I imagine parts of my story may feel familiar to you, no matter what your race or ethnicity. If you have gone through the seemingly endless quest to have a child, you know the struggle. Sharing stories, it becomes clear that infertility enrolls you in a sisterhood you never wanted to join. The commonality is that we all have slightly different versions of the same story. My personal opinion is that as women we share a collective experience of super-hero syndrome. We are powerful beings, we want to do it all and we tend to suffer alone. As infertile women, or women who have been devastated by a pregnancy loss, we share a common pain. If you happen to be a woman of color, your isolation is unique. Infertility, like any disease, does not discriminate as to whom it will touch. Yet, when we begin to share our stories, the discrimination is revealed in the narratives that do not hold space for women of color. We have never truly been a part of the discussion, our needs have never really been addressed, and it is time to start shifting that narrative and sharing the larger space.

Everyone deserves the chance to have their story told. Centering the story on the experiences of women of color allows us inclusion in a world dominated by stories told from one perspective: affluent, white, and heteronormative. You would never even know women of color exist in this space. You certainly don't see us in news articles or

1   A. Chandra et al. "Infertility and Impaired Fecundity in the United States, 1982-2010: Data From the National Survey of Family Growth," *National Health Statistics Reports*, 67, (2013): 1-19, accessed February 7, 2018, https://www.cdc.gov/nchs/data/nhsr/nhsr067.pdf

2   Melissa F. Wellons et al. "Racial Differences in Self-Reported Infertility and Risk Factors for Infertility in a Cohort of Black and White Women: The CARDIA Women's Study," *Fertil Steril*, 90, no. 5, (2008): 1640-48, https://www.ncbi.nlm.nih.gov/pmc/articles/PMC2592196

on TV, on magazine covers, or on posters or pamphlets in medical waiting rooms. Instead, we are inundated with the same types of images of a white woman fawning over her miracle baby. Those are very real stories, but they aren't the only stories, and they're not representative of all the women who have struggled and fought for the privilege of being called "mother." For centuries, women of color have been sidelined to bear witness to the stories of others. We struggle to advocate for ourselves because we are not listened to and we are marginalized within a system that was never set up to support us. When you look in the mirror and don't see yourself reflected back, you start to believe that your experience is not valid, but that's not true. As the authors of *Silent and Infertile* write: "Overall, when black women could not conceive a child, it negatively affected their self-esteem. They saw themselves as abnormal, in part, because they did not see other people like themselves—African-American, female, and infertile—in social images."[3] We can't sit back and allow other people to own our stories anymore. We are real. Our stories are real. What we experience is real, and our voices deserve to be heard. The pain of infertility has no racial boundaries but women of color are unfairly burdened by prejudice and bias within medical systems. We have to navigate within a world where access to care, treatment, and financial support have negative effects on health outcomes. Historically and culturally, the trope of the Black woman is associated with abundance and hyper-fertility. As Regina Townsend, author of the blog *The Broken Brown Egg*, is quoted as saying, "With women of color, specifically Hispanic and African-American women, the stigma attached to us is that it's not hard to have kids, and that we have a lot of kids... And when you're the

---

3   Rosario Ceballo, Erin T. Graham, Jamie Hart, "Silent and Infertile: An Intersectional Analysis of the Experiences of Socioeconomically Diverse African American Women With Infertility," *Psychology of Women Quarterly*, 39, no. 4 (2015): 497-511

one who can't, you feel like, 'I've failed.'"[4] The reality is bleak and stark. Women of color are twice as likely to be infertile, have lower implantation and pregnancy success rates, have increased probability of miscarriage, and, most devastating of all, face the highest maternal death rates in the industrial world.[5] For Asian women, the outcomes are also different from the status quo and the medical field seems uninterested in understanding why. Infertility studies are primarily focused on Caucasian women. One of the few people researching women of color is Dr. Victor Fujimoto, Director of the IVF program at the University of California, San Francisco. He found that, "When looking at our population of Asian patients, 40 percent or more were delayed in speaking for at least two years after their problem began"[6] The article about him goes on to say, "He also found that Asian American women have 33 percent lower successful pregnancy rates after IVF treatment compared to Caucasian women."[7] Hispanic women can face the very same cultural stigma that Black and Asian communities share. Cultural biases may be a strong deterrent to seeking out fertility treatments. For women that are Native American, First Nations, or Indigenous Peoples, there are no major studies to even pull information from regarding infertility. How can we address the issue and provide support to our sisters when they are literally not seen or counted? Medical bias against minority groups can lead to health disparity that determines how women of color get diagnosed and treated. Not only do minority women have to contend with the trauma of in-

4   Tanzina Vega, "Infertility, Endured Through a Prism of Race," *New York Times*, April 25, 2014, https://www.nytimes.com/2014/04/26/us/infertility-endured-through-a-prism-of-race.html.

5   Amy Roeder, "America is Failing Its Black Mothers," *Harvard Public Health*, Winter 2019, https://www.hsph.harvard.edu/magazine/magazine_article/america-is-failing-its-black-mothers

6   Tommy Na, "Is Asian Infertility a Thing?" *Mochi Magazine*, September 27, 2019, https://mochimag.com/lifestyle/health/is-asian-fertility-a-thing

7   Na, "Is Asian Infertility a Thing?"

fertility, but we also have to establish trust within a system that does not support our infertility diagnosis and treatment needs.

So, where do we go from here? In recognizing the feelings of women of color as they navigate infertility: I hope you find resilience, strength, hope, and the resources that help. While celebrities speaking out helps to normalize and take away the stigma of infertility and treatment, many people desperately need to hear stories and find community with regular women out of the spotlight. No matter where you are in your story––if you're currently experiencing infertility, if you've come out through the other side, if you have a child, if you're adopting, if you're grieving a loss––you are a survivor. Being a survivor is about reclaiming your power. Your story does not have to be complete for you to find resolution and peace.

The hardest thing for me to accept about my infertility was coming to terms with the fact that I was completely out of control. I lost control of everything: my body, my schedule, my sex life, my daily decisions. It is also realizing that even with all the advanced medical technology and new ways of making a baby, at the end of it all, it comes down to blind luck. So, if motherhood is your dream, what happens when you find out that your dream won't be coming true? How do you begin to redefine your greatest hope and still have it all make sense?

This book is an open conversation. It is about the long, hard, twisted journey we take as we dream of becoming mothers. It was not enough for me to simply tell my story, it felt critical to share the stories of others as well. Women of color, in their words and in their way, openly share their experiences in this book. I would only say two things to the women I interviewed: The first was, "Begin where you want to begin in your story," and the second was, "What advice would you give to yourself if you could go back and do it all over again?" An interview expected to take twenty minutes would often last for two hours. There were many tears, there were a few laughs, and sometimes there was a lot of swearing, but every woman wanted to give voice to their experience to help someone else.

Make no mistake, infertility is traumatic. There is no way to shortcut through the struggle, grief, loss, or pain. You have to allow yourself to move through it to come out on the other side. What I will say is that at least now I know I'm not alone. I hope you know that you're not alone either.

Chapter One

INFERTILITY:

Why is it so Hard to Get Knocked Up?

"What screws us up the most in life is the picture in our head of what it's supposed to be."

-Jeremy Binns

W hat do you do if your perception of your world gets turned upside down? As one popular song puts it, how do you breathe when there is no air? If you are in this fight—and trust me, it can feel like a massive battle between you and your body—you know there are two opposing realities: Infertility means having to acknowledge both the beauty of the dream of motherhood and also the shock of the cruel specter of childlessness.

We all know the dream. Some small details may vary, but it is all basically the same if you grow up seeing yourself as one day becoming a mother. The dream is so beautiful, it feels comically (and almost cruelly) easy to attain; you get pregnant, carry the baby, have the baby, and get to live out your version of motherhood. Getting pregnant should be the easy (and fun) part. A mere preamble to the cool mom sorority of late-night feedings, diapers, Mommy & Me classes, and playground playdates. Any tears you shed on the path to motherhood are tears of joy. There are tears at the positive pregnancy test, the sonograms, and the wondrous time-stopping moment when you hear that first cry. Everyone lives happily ever after. For a woman dealing with infertility, the harsh, exhausting reality is it's hard, painful (mentally, physically, and emotionally), and plain sucks. It's not fair. It's not your fault, yet you somehow feel an overwhelming responsibility. Your body is no longer yours. Your cycles are manipulated, you are poked and prodded in the most invasive ways, your eggs are counted, your hormones are monitored, your blood is taken, and you endure daily shots. All of that is on a good day. There isn't a simple solution to any of the choices presented and childbirth is less of a miracle and more of a carefully engineered scientific event. Surgeries, pills, shots: they can all "fix" things, but even getting pregnant or having a baby does not cure all the pain, heartbreak, and discomfort that came before. In the end, it takes a lot of luck, hope, and the true miracle is that somehow we are all left standing at the end of the day, trying to find some peace to calm all the crazy that swirls around us.

Infertility comes with a flood of emotions (none of them positive). You may find that you are angry and sad simultaneously. The one reaction that may surprise you the most is how it utterly destroys your dream. It's that sting—that feeling of being cheated out of something that *should* come naturally—and having to sit and watch others effortlessly obtain the thing that you yearn for most of all. That perfect version of the life that you had envisioned for yourself is suddenly gone and you are left feeling whiplashed. Getting pregnant loses its beauty and gets lost in a chore of timetables, charts, shots, hormone therapy, and treatments. Trying to have a baby becomes hard work—none of it is enjoyable. If you are lucky enough to get pregnant, just being pregnant is no longer a time of bliss, celebration, and joy. Every doctor's appointment or sonogram brings hope mixed with a dose of fear. If you are facing infertility, the blissful dream of pregnancy can feel like a nightmare. The clinical diagnosis of infertility hits home, straight to your core. Infertility is simply the inability to reproduce by natural means; there is nothing simple in how that diagnosis can make you feel. I felt that my body had betrayed me. My body could not live up to its most momentous biological task. All of a sudden, my diagnosis had revealed my worst enemy: me. I had to battle my body to achieve my dream. How do you begin a fight if you love and have spent a lifetime caring for your enemy? You "kill" it with kindness. I had always taken care of my body; I worked out, did yoga, and ate right. That was the most frustrating thing. I felt like I had done everything right up to that point. How do I make sense of the fact that none of that mattered? I wasn't just infertile, I was broken and it wasn't going to be an easy fix.

It left me in a very lonely place. In 2010, I didn't know anyone else who was infertile. Sure, I had read a couple of *People Magazine* stories about a celebrity or two and their "difficulty" getting pregnant, but in real life, as far as I knew, I was the only one.

♥ ♡ ♥

NO, NO, NO
By: Tisha

I was in shock. I was staring at the doctor's mouth and I knew he was saying things but I only heard my own voice in my head screaming *NO*. I was in complete disbelief. *I need help getting pregnant? Are you crazy? Are you out of your mind? What are you talking about?* Obviously, my doctor had mixed up my test results with someone else. I'm fine.

My internal monologue began with the easy fix. *Well, if there is something wrong, why can't you just give me a pill to regulate my periods? My co-worker just needed a pill, and she was pregnant in a month.* From there, it went to shame. *Why me? I must have done something wrong. This is somehow my fault.* I even said to myself, *I think my husband should have been wearing boxers and not briefs.* Then, it quickly shifted to sadness. *Why is everyone else getting pregnant so easily? Why not me? I want to have a baby so much; it's so unfair.* Then the full reality hit of what it meant to be diagnosed with infertility—the money! *I can't believe how much this is going to cost.*

The cost of infertility is daunting for most women. Communities of color are especially impacted by finances. My past infertility nurse even told me that they lose more minority patients due to finances than for any other reason. Women of color are often diagnosed with infertility later or misdiagnosed—that costs money. We face underlying problems like fibroids that need to be addressed before infertility treatments. Again, this requires more money. I had insurance that covered infertility and let me tell you, we blew through that coverage before we even reached the first transfer cycle. All told, the thousands and thousands of dollars we spent trying to get pregnant was not money that we had lying around. We were lucky to have amazing parents that were extremely supportive. My mother-in-law and my mom were willing to do anything to help my husband and I have their grandchild. Even with that help, we got very creative in finding ways to cover all the costs.

IT WASN'T A VACATION

By: Ash

The tide is beginning to come in. A slow rise, not strong and unruly like the Atlantic. Incredibly clear, ombré aquamarine waters. Palm trees, white sands. Me and my honey resting, laughing, sharing bits of our reading materials or the earphones. A great vacation. Except it's not. The vacation atmosphere is a much-needed secondary benefit, but not at all the decisive factor. I thought there would be more people of my phenotype here. In fact, there was only one donor in the program who was a phenotype match. One. But this program is much cheaper. Significantly. To the extent that it cannot be ignored. It was the decisive factor. I really wanted to continue with my reproductive endocrinologist, I was comfortable with her practice and her care providers. It's kind of weird to think that this part of the journey is without them. But, the cost!

So, here we are.

We had hoped for a minimum of six to eight eggs. We got three. *Do we cancel? Are the odds against us? Do we find a new donor?* As said, there was only one compatible donor in the program, so we would have to go to a US egg bank. We did not have the funds to acquire new eggs. But, new considerations began to emerge. Going into this process, I had several concerns with egg donation. One: women don't naturally produce multiple eggs, two at most. Oocyte donation, unlike sperm donation for men, is taxing. I did not want someone to suffer harm because I wanted a baby. Two: we want a family but not a basketball team! *Would we fertilize all the eggs? What would we do with extra embryos?* Three: if God bestows us with twins, we will be overjoyed, but we do not want to fabricate twins. I am small and old. One embryo at a time, please!

♥ ♡ ♥

It is not easy to get women, regardless of color, to open up about infertility. If you are living in it right now, it can be hard to see the light at the end of the tunnel. If you have moved on to a different place in life, revisiting the pain can be daunting. In all my years of leading and sharing in support groups and advocacy efforts, I always use this simple exercise to begin the conversation: "Fill in the blanks: Infertility is . . ." and more often than not, with that simple introduction the door is opened. What has stood out over the years is how similar the feelings of frustration, exhaustion, and sadness are among the answers I receive.

"Overwhelming, disappointing, emotional, expensive, exhausting."

"A *never-ending* battle that *sometimes* gets the best of me and makes me feel defeated."

"Like a sentence for a crime you didn't commit."

"The thief of my life."

"Exhausting."

"Sucks, makes you doubt yourself, makes you question everything."

"Painful, not fair, heartbreaking, stressful, embarrassing, shameful, depressing, empty."

"More common than you realize."

"Heartbreaking."

"An ongoing curse that takes away your youth, your hope, your joy, your dreams that you made that will never come true without some far-fetched miracle."

Finally, my favorite, which I came across in an unknown-authored meme and it sums it all up perfectly, "Infertility (n) a medical condition which diminishes self-esteem, your social life as well as checking and savings accounts. Causes sudden urges to pee on a stick, cry or scream, and a fear of pregnancy announcements. Treated by medical professionals who you pay to knock you up. This does not always work. Affects 1 in 10 couples."

I FELT LOST

By: Alicia

It's difficult to convey the emotion, the sense of helplessness, regret, and distress that infertility brought to my world. I cannot adequately describe the failing faith, the doubt, and the faltering steps, or the resignation that became so commonplace to my everyday thinking.

In 2007, I was in my mid-thirties and on a work assignment in Kenya. I was at the age when I had assumed I would have a family and did not—that age when your mind and spirit begin to nudge towards worry, but your psyche tells you it will all be alright. The mind is so protective. Rehashing all the "should-ofs" and "could-ofs" serves no purpose. Many of the Kenyans with whom I happened to talk about family, like so many other non-Western European cultures, believed in finding your mate young and having children. I was, as one said, "cursed," as evidenced by my lack of marriage and children. I was, as another said, "fortunate with resources and opportunities" and so should adopt—clearly, this was God's calling for me as I had no children. I recalled my father telling me just a few months earlier that, having bought a home, I was now no longer marriageable. What man would want a wife who could already provide for herself? I remember a friend of my mom's congratulating me for obtaining two graduate degrees and then expressing her regrets that as a Black woman I was now among those unlikely to ever wed. Later, back in the US, a stranger on the tram asked if I had children and then urged me to go ahead and admit that I did not want any, saying "it's ok to admit it." (Really, what do you say in such a moment, to a stranger, in such a public place?) I remember a lady in Bible study class telling me that since it had not yet happened, that it was not God's plan and I needed to consider what else God was calling me to. (Why do people speak as if they have the commission and authority of God?). Any one of these statements taken in isolation were fine—they rolled off my back like water off a duck. But after years of this, and their seeming truth as I had not gotten married and did not have children, they had a cumulative effect of convincing me that maybe I really was cursed and that God really had forsaken me.

Finding out I was infertile, I had to let go of that hope of ever carrying a child myself. That was a hard dream to let go of; it reset my life. I am not exaggerating when I say that I mourned in the same way I would mourn the death of a loved one. I grieved the loss of everything I thought my life would be and had to accept that my perfect dream living in my head was never going to happen. Infertility hit me so hard that it felt like a full-force punch in the gut. I wasn't totally naive. I knew there would be some kind of issue with getting pregnant. A diagnosis usually comes after you have been trying unsuccessfully to get pregnant for a year, or if you are over thirty-five, after six months. I had been diagnosed with endometriosis when I was in college and had undergone three surgeries for that condition. I was thirty-seven and fully understood that age could necessitate some kind of intervention. Whatever I imagined, I did not see my life becoming completely consumed by having a child. I didn't even have an inkling that soon every waking moment would be spent doing everything imaginable to get pregnant. In Vitro Fertilization (IVF) wasn't even on my radar. Did I even know what IVF stood for? I thought that maybe I would get a shot and be fine. When I went to the doctor after six months of trying, I knew there would be tests, but I assumed that the end remedy would be simple. After hearing my history, my OB-GYN sent me to have a test that would determine if, or to what extent, my tubes were blocked. The hysterosalpingogram (HSG) test is done by injecting a harmless dye into the womb and monitoring its flow into the fallopian tubes. For me, this test was excruciatingly painful. I didn't understand why at the time. I was left crying and writhing on the exam table for the duration of the test. Later I found out the reason the HSG was so painful was because the tech kept pumping in more and more dye to unblock the tubes and the pressure was building up with nowhere to go. Whatever was blocking my tubes was not moving. Two days later I got a phone call from my doctor; it was the call that altered my life: "Candace, both your tubes are blocked. Your only option to get pregnant is to go right to IVF. I can't help you. I am going to have to refer you to a specialist." There it was—the gut punch. How was I supposed to unpack the raw and bitter reality of everything the doctor just said? It was like falling down the rabbit hole and hitting my head on every protruding rock on the way down.

Both tubes are blocked—BAM!

You have to do IVF—BAM!

I can't help you—BAM!

I was devastated. I didn't see the light at the end of the tunnel, I saw the tunnel blocked and dark at both ends, just like my tubes. IVF was foreign to me at that time. I wasn't sure what it was, but knew that it was going to be expensive and intimidating. I had so many questions, yet I couldn't find a way to voice any of them. I told my husband and saw on his face the confusion and fear that I had in my head. I was lost, alone, angry, and deeply ashamed. No one I knew was infertile. Certainly, no black women. If I had any certainty at that point, it was the certainty that I was alone.

There it is, the painful truth. All the images, the stories, the pictures, the magazine covers: everything I knew about infertility told me that it did not affect anyone who resembled me. Not only was I going to be forced to live in the pain of my diagnosis, but I was also going to be living in my pain all alone. Today, I know that women of color are the real silent majority of infertility, and I know how common miscarriage is during pregnancy. But on that day in 2010, when I found out that I wouldn't be able to get pregnant without a lot of intervention, the only thing I knew for sure was that I felt uniquely by myself in what was about to happen. As discussed by Arianna Davis and Robin Hilmantel, "Infertility affects at least 12 percent of all women up to the age of forty-four, and studies suggest Black women may be almost twice as likely to experience infertility as white women. Yet only about eight percent of Black women between the ages of twenty-five and forty-four seek medical help to get pregnant, compared to fifteen percent of white women. It begs the question: Why isn't there more conversation about Black women and infertility?"[1]

---

1   Ariana Davis and Robin Hilmantel, "This is Why We Chose to Talk About Black Women and Infertility," *Women's Health Magazine*, October 2018.   https://www.womenshealthmag.com/health/a23785945/black-women-infertility-letter-from-the-editors

♥ ♡ ♥

THERE IS A STIGMA

By: Dr. Theresa Buckson, OB-GYN

Honestly, the biggest obstacle women of color often face is the stigma of being infertile. When you are ashamed, it is that much harder to seek out treatment or support. A number of my patients in the beginning are in total denial—they feel as if there is no way that they can be infertile. No one ever really discusses it in the Black community. Issues like fibroids, PCOS, and endometriosis really impact the health of Black women and many of my patients are not prepared for that.

It has gotten better. In 2010 when my infertility journey began, Michelle Obama had not come forward with her infertility experience. Gabrielle Union had not yet undergone her journey to motherhood through surrogacy. Beyoncé had not yet been pregnant and openly shared her struggles. We are at a point where Tyra Banks, Tamaron Hall, Mariah Carey, Chrissy Teigan, and so many more women of color have shared with us their pregnancy struggles. They have helped kick down the door of secrecy, shame, and isolation. Representation is real. After the former First Lady opened up about using IVF to conceive her daughters, and Gabrielle Union detailed her road to surrogacy, some fertility centers saw an increase of almost 20 percent in women of color seeking treatment.[2]

---

2   Katie Kindelan, "Michelle Obama effect' sees more black women seeking fertility treatment 1 year after 'Becoming,'" *Good Morning America Website,* December 17, 2019. https://www.goodmorningamerica.com/wellness/story/michelle-obama-effect-sees-black-women-seeking-fertility-67685029

Still, the prevailing narrative of infertility remains: white, affluent, and heteronormative. As author Belle Boggs says, "This image is so common that many doctors have internalized the stereotype, assuming that white women are most at risk for infertility. This misperception can affect research, referrals to reproductive endocrinologists, and outreach to potential patients."[3] So, representation matters, not only for treatment, but for diagnosis before treatment even begins. The diagnosis alone will knock you off your axis, no matter how prepared you think you are. If you add all of that into navigating a system that is unprepared to address your needs, your options may feel insurmountable. The importance of people in the public eye coming forward is that the struggles of minority women become part of the conversation and when you are part of the conversation, you can start to affect change. As Rachel Leah states, "Both Obama and Union are helping to break the code of silence that's a symptom of the cultural shame cast on women who struggle with 'normal' pregnancy, a standard too often prescribed as essential to womanhood, which relegates so many to the margins, including women who are infertile, disabled, transgender, or who don't want to have children. But it's particularly powerful for Union and Obama to be cultivating these conversations with the public—by doing so, they are helping to create space for women of color, and Black women especially, to be at the center of these issues. This is a particularly radical endeavor when you take note of who is traditionally centered in conversations about infertility, and more importantly, who is typically left out."[4]

---

3   Belle Boggs, "The Significance of Michelle Obama's Fertility Story," *The Atlantic*, November 14, 2018. https://www.theatlantic.com/family/archive/2018/11/michelle-obamas-ivf-story-means-lot-black-women/575824

4   Rachel Leah, "Why Gabrielle Union and Michelle Obama opening up about miscarriage and infertility matters," *Salon*, December 12, 2018. https://www.salon.com/2018/12/12/why-gabrielle-union-and-michelle-obama-opening-up-about-miscarriage-and-infertility-matters

My diagnosis felt like the death of a dream, but my husband likes to remind me that it is more like having a different version of the dream. It is not about giving birth to a baby, it has always been about having a family. The best advice we ever received from our doctor was to come up for air now and then and re-examine our goals. Realizing that success is something we could define for ourselves, it opened us up to a world where there is no right way to form a family. There is a way that works for you. We get to define our success in our story. But all in all, infertility sucks, there is no way around that. It just sucks. So, I am so sorry if you are going through it and I hope you are consoled as you define this new version of your dream.

REFLECTION

*"Never underestimate the
power of hope."*

-Unknown

With stories that dive deep into internal pain and sadness, it can be very easy to miss the thing they all have in common—hope. All the stories, even the ones that express the most frustration, are grounded in the eternally optimistic sense of hope. Infertility is overwhelming, yet we still have hope. Infertility steals your life, yet we still have hope. Infertility sucks in every way, every day, and still, we cling to the hope that it will work out for us. We think, why not? We could be part of that successful group. We could get pregnant. There is a possibility. There is power in the resilience it takes to not lose hope. I know the popular and conventional thing to say is that if you could do it all over again, you wouldn't change a thing. People also love to say that everything happens for a reason or that what you are going through is part of a grand plan. I look back and think that there are a million things I would have done differently. I am not angry or sad at the decisions I made, I just think of what could have been different and then think about how that could have changed the outcome. That is the beauty of hindsight. Looking back at where you were and being able to see clearly in a way that you could not when you were in the fog and emotionally invested in every minute detail. I now know that I wasn't ready to start the process of adoption when I first found out I was infertile. I know I wasn't ready to even talk about the possibility of donor eggs until after I had more than one failed cycle. I didn't think that I would keep trying after a miscarriage. Moving through all of that brought me to where I am today: a happy (and exhausted) mom.

Everyone's experience will lead to a different outcome and there is no shame in deciding to bow out at any point along the way. It's important to affirm one another and not judge anyone else's experience or emotions that may be different from our own. As my six-year-old likes to say, "Don't yuck someone's yum." There are a million reasons that you make the choices you make and all of them are valid. You did not do anything to deserve infertility. Infertility happened to you and it is not fair, but you will be OKAY. Nothing about this is easy, but you have support (more on that later) and no matter how it all ends up, you will come out on the other side. Your happiness is not tied to any specific outcome. You get to define your life and you don't have to explain your choices to anybody.

Chapter One acknowledges that there is no right way to form a family. The way that works for you forms your definition of success. The road to creating a family probably looks nothing like what you planned. Let's also acknowledge that sometimes success may look like the resolution of living child-free. Circumstance may lead you down a road where success is an end to an emotionally, physically, and exhausting journey. In one of my last appointments with the Reproductive Endocrinologist (RE), I had to face the reality that living child-free was a real possibility. I was down to two frozen embryos (not the best grade), and none of us had any confidence that the embryos would stick at the next transfer, or that I would have success with the surrogate I had chosen. The meeting was so bleak that my RE broke down and cried. Yes, you read that correctly—I broke my RE. A man whose life's work involved infertile patients; a physician, who was at the top of his field and had probably delivered sad news to thousands of couples that they were nearing the end of this particular journey. We were the couple that broke him. My husband and I left the office and we cried. Then we had a real heart-to-heart talk about what our life would be like without kids. Not the casual "what if" conversation, the serious one. The one where you start looking at budgets, new jobs, and new places to live. We talked through what our life would really look like. We imagined leaving Los Angeles and my husband transferring to New York for work. We imagined decorating the incredibly cool apartment we would have on the Upper West Side, all the exotic vacations we would take, and the restaurants we would visit unhampered by parenthood. We invested time in reimagining and redefining our life. It was going to be a good life, just the two of us. The story could have ended there, but we weren't ready to give up our dream of being parents, we had to redefine what success would look like. Our journey to parenthood was not going to end with me being pregnant and having a child. We would not give up, but we had to move forward to a new reality and new life. If we wanted to be parents, we had to be open to finding a different way to make it happen.

Chapter Two

THE DIAGNOSIS:
Why is this Happening to Me?

*"No one prepares you for the hate
you feel for yourself because your
body just can't do what it was meant
to do . . . "*

-Unknown

No matter how much we try to prepare for our life, we are never equipped to handle most of the sudden pitfalls. Infertility is never your story until it is YOUR story. No one is ready to hear that they are infertile or that they might need help. That fateful day I found out I was infertile, when the doctor was patiently explaining to me all the test results and the options, all I heard was "blah, blah, blah . . . you can't have a baby." That was the moment, during that call, that my life became an out-of-control blur. I spent the next four years feeling like I was slowly being drowned in a sea of needles, tests, estrogen patches, shots, pills, transfers, surgeries, two-week waits, and pregnancy tests. I spent more time and money peeing on sticks than I spent getting myself up and dressed in the morning. It was a bleak truth. At thirty-eight, I was of advanced maternal age. That alone, without any other contributing factors, seemed to condemn me into the abyss of infertility.

There is a vast difference between expectation and reality. My husband Tommaso and I are a couple of the new millennium. In our thirties, we were each divorced from the "starter marriage" of our twenties. We met on Match.com and our first major conversations took place over several weeks of email. Our first date was supposed to be a carefully curated forty-five minutes at a trendy West Hollywood coffee shop where we would have a polite and non-threatening first-date conversation. That was the expectation. The reality . . . being a new transplant to Los Angeles from San Francisco, and it being the days before every car came equipped with navigation, and it being 5 pm in Los Angeles rush-hour traffic, I got hopelessly lost. It took me three hours to find my way to meet Tommaso for our first date and he stayed on the phone trying to help me most of the time. So what should have been a quick meet-and-greet was now a two-martini pizza dinner. Our conversation was a belly-laugh inducing, bonding discussion about all the horrible Match.com dates we had endured. Our first kiss was in a parking lot—while the setting was not romantic, the sentiment was, in every way. That was in June. I moved in with him in September and a year and a half later we were married on a beach in Maui in front of twenty-four of our most loved friends and family.

At thirty-eight, with a history of endometriosis and fibroids, I was savvy enough to know that getting pregnant might not be easy. I never thought I wouldn't get pregnant, I just thought it would take a bit of time and planning. I wasn't the only one with those thoughts. As soon as I got engaged, my mom and mother-in-law bonded together, called me, and flat out said that I was no spring chicken. I was advised by these culturally traditional women that I shouldn't worry about waiting for the wedding. They wanted their grandchild right away! So, that was the plan. I even spent a considerable amount of time trying to find a maternity wedding dress and planned on making the gender reveal at the reception before we cut the cake. It was going to be so perfect.

The wedding was beautiful. By that time, we had realized that something was wrong but we chalked it up to a couple of different things: Maybe we were having sex on the wrong days, so we made a chart. Maybe I miscalculated my ovulation, so we started doing an at-home test. Maybe I had to change my diet or lose weight. Maybe he was wearing the wrong underwear and not keeping his sperm cool. Maybe we had to try a specific position or I had to put a pillow under my butt afterward. Don't laugh—I am sure you tried everything too before you had to face the fact that you needed a little bit of outside intervention.

BLINDSIDED

By: Lola

I'm forty-two and, starting last year, my partner and I were like, "Okay, well, let's try for another one." I'm okay either way, if we only have our one or if we have more kids. But, it would be nice to have a sibling for our son. So, when we went to a family doctor, and I mentioned to her that yeah, I was trying again—we weren't being super serious or disciplined about it but we were trying—the doctor was like, "Okay. So how old are you?" She looked at my age and her first response to seeing I was over forty was, "Okay, well, we work with this fertility specialist." I was like, "What?" I was very shocked that fertility was something that needed to be talked about. Infertility was never on my radar. On social media, people have their own platforms and stuff but even in those conversations, I think I might have seen one Asian woman who couldn't get pregnant despite trying but that's it. Nothing besides that was on my radar when it came to Asian women and infertility. I did call the doctor and say, "Okay, fine, connect us with the fertility clinic." I didn't think it was anything that we needed to discuss, but as soon as you're over forty, that's it. It's a thing. Maybe six months from now I will be like, "Oh crap, I am going through this." Infertility is here. Asian families (like mine) don't do feelings. That's where a lot of problems happen as adults because we weren't given that opportunity to dive into the emotional side of our being and that's the most important side. I'm sure if I share my fertility issues with my mom, I'm sure she would just play it down. It would be like, "Well, whatever. If it doesn't happen, it doesn't happen" . . . yeah, move on kind of thing.

With all the problems I had growing up, I feel like I shouldn't have been surprised to find out I was infertile. It all started badly and it never really got better. When I was twelve, I started my period. I also started my thirty-five-year battle with debilitating endometriosis (although I wouldn't officially be diagnosed with this disease and treated for it until I was twenty-one). My pain and discomfort were so intense at twelve that I would beg to stay home from school if I was having my period. My parents and my doctor told me that all women have cramps and that I should take some Advil. When I told my doctor that when I had cramps, I could only get some relief by taking four or five Advil at a time, he looked at me and casually said that's way too much, try taking only two. I wasn't just ignored, I was dismissed. I knew something was wrong, my body did not feel right. My pain level was through the roof. Yet I was consistently told by doctors that what I was feeling was normal. Again and again, I was told that all women have cramps. I have never understood why we, as women, often accept that pain and discomfort are an accepted part of our lives.

I spent my entire young life thinking that my monthly pain and heavy flow were completely normal. It wasn't until I was in college and living in a dorm that I began to be aware that other girls were not paralyzed in bed during their cycle. Other girls were not spending their periods nauseous, vomiting, and going through Ultra Plus Size Tampax at a rate of three to four an hour for days on end. Other girls were not passing large blood clots. Everything I thought was normal about my period experience was turned on its head.

At twenty-one, I started looking for doctors who would perform a hysterectomy on me; I had no idea about endometriosis, I only knew that I could not survive decades of the pain on a monthly basis. I was ready and willing, in college, to stop the pain by the most permanent means available. I never found a willing doctor, but I did find a doctor who said it sounded like endometriosis and he would do laparoscopic surgery to confirm this and remove any endometrial tissue. When I woke up from surgery, all I remember is the doctor confirming that I did indeed have endometriosis. He told me later that in my post-surgery drug haze, I smiled the biggest smile he had seen and said to him, "YES! I knew something was wrong!" After years of being told that all my pain was in my head, or wasn't that bad, or wasn't a big deal, I had confirmation that something had been wrong inside me all along. I never imagined that being diagnosed with a disease would be so joyously validating. For the first time, I felt that since I knew the exact problem, I finally had something specific to fix. Of course, I didn't know then that I would spend the next quarter-century of my life trying to fix it all (endometriosis and fibroids are a lifetime commitment to pain). All I knew was that at twenty-one, I thought I had all the answers.

I WISH I FOUGHT HARDER

By: Sandra

Twenty-one years of pain with Endo (before officially being diagnosed). Nine plus years of infertility. I wish I fought harder for my health.

Because of Endo, I cannot have children naturally. Because of Endo, my egg reserve is low. Because of Endo, I am premenopausal at thirty-seven. I wish I fought harder to be heard. I wish I knew more about this disease back then.

Even though it may be too late for me, it is not for you. I will use my voice to fight for you. I will fight for Endometriosis, Adenomyosis, PCOS, Uterine Fibroids, and Infertility. Your pain is NOT normal. Keep fighting.

♥ ♡ ♥

IT ALL STARTED WITH A PERIOD

By: Halima | Founder and President of FemCare

I am a woman of color who came here as a refugee, who was born to abusive parents, and was also raised as a Muslim woman. I'm no longer Muslim, I'm a Born-again Christian, but I had a terrible experience when it came to my period. My introduction to getting my period was intense. I had my period in my aunt's house, and when I came home my father laughed at me, shaming me in front of my entire family. It got worse after that. I was abused for getting my period, I had endometriosis, and I also lived with

premenstrual deport disorder—I had the symptoms for a long time and didn't get diagnosed
until I was about twenty-eight years old. When
I tell my story, I start to tear up. I get so angry
because I feel like the people who were supposed to take care of me and make sure that I
had a good experience didn't . . . and that they
made it worse. So it makes me angry, even when
I think about how I was bullied a lot in school.
I was one of the first girls to get my period and
so the other girls teased me because I was different. I had something they didn't and they bullied
me instead of supporting me through it. I think
a lot of that had to do with their lack of education. If they had education and understood that
periods come at different ages for different girls,
then they would've known that there's no need
to be jealous because everyone's going to get it.
We should support each other through this, but
nothing like that ever happened to me.

This is how I found out I had endometriosis:
I was working as a nurse and one day I was in ex-
treme pain. Even though I had taken three Advil
Extra Strength before I went to work, I was in agony. I was trying to open a package and I couldn't
because my hands were shaking because I was in
so much pain. It got to a point where I couldn't
even administer medications anymore because of
the pain. I thought, *Why am I doing this to myself? I'm dying and in pain right now, I need to
leave.* So I locked my medication cart and I went
to my colleague and I said, "I need to leave." My
colleague said, "Halima, what's wrong with you?
Your lips are purple." When I looked at my face,
my lips were purple and my face was grey. I had
no color left. I looked like I was dying. I was

shaking. Imagine, even with all of that, because I was living in poverty, I didn't take a taxi home, I walked home because I wanted to save money. I didn't have that much money, I was already only working as a part-time nurse to begin with, so I walked home in all that pain. I got home, took three more Advil and two Percocet. That was when I realized this is not normal. I didn't sleep that night. The pain literally would not stop—it was indescribable. To this day, thank the Lord, it's never been that bad again. It was non-stop for twenty-four hours. So I finally had to go to the ER and get an IV drip because the pain was so intense. That's what it took—only the IV drip stopped the pain. Can you believe that? That's when I went to my doctor and I said, "I'm not leaving this office until you send me to a specialist to find out what's going on with me because I've been coming to you for ten years now with pain. You keep saying, it's nothing, it's nothing, it's nothing. Now send me to find out what's going on." And as it turned out, I had endometriosis, which was diagnosed by a gynecologist who told me with a smile on her face that I probably wasn't going to be able to have kids.

I'm just angry now. I don't feel sadness—I don't feel it. I'm just angry. But I'm also intentional with my anger. I'm like, "Okay, I'm angry, and so now I'm going to use this anger to advocate for myself, to become an aggressive self-advocate. I don't care what I have to do to make sure that my health and well-being is prioritized. I will do it." Another thing people have told me is that if I have kids, the pain will stop, which is so dehumanizing. So, I should have a kid so my period cramps stop? And you wonder why this world is so messed up. I am not here to break the cycle; I am here, telling my story, to break the wheel.

♥ ♡ ♥

I TRIED TO DO EVERYTHING "RIGHT"

By: Maya

This takes me back because it was such a confusing time. I'm forty now and we started trying when I was thirty. So, it's been a decade. I did yoga and acupuncture, ate all the right things, gave up coffee, and I'm healthy. So, we had a "plan" for how it was all going to go. We started trying and after six months, I was like, what's going on here?

I'm a "type A" person who gets things done. Why can't I get this done? I went to an OB, and I think it was really unfortunate that he just didn't have infertility experience, so he didn't do a lot of testing. He tested my FSH and then he was like, "Well, you're healthy—just keep on trucking." So, I lost almost two years in that process. I eventually did Clomid and that was traumatizing. In all my years of meds, I feel like Clomid was the hardest. I felt batshit crazy! And even after all that, the doctor never checked my tubes. Now, if you don't have tubes that work, you can't get sperm to where it needs to go. When my tubes were finally checked, I had some problems with one of them. I was not educated enough on any of this.

I think that is such a big piece for all women to understand. Women need to educate themselves so that we can advocate for ourselves! We need to understand ovarian reserve and what parts need to be in working order to make trying to conceive even an option. Because if we don't know these things, we're just following the lead of somebody else. On paper, and physically, I looked fine. I was told, "You're thirty-two, you've got ovaries, you get your period, you're going to be all right here." Then suddenly my life started this descent into the abyss of fertility struggle. I think that is somewhat common for people who struggle when they're under the age of thirty-five. When the Fertility Specialist did extensive testing, his face went from: oh great, I've got a thirty-two-year-old, I can get in and out with a couple of IUI's or one round of IVF or whatever he might have been thinking to having to tell me, at thirty-two, that I had diminished ovarian reserve and now we have big problems. It was very confusing to me.

Why? What caused that? How did that happen? There aren't a lot of answers, just more and more questions, and I feel like that's such a hard thing even when you do have a diagnosis. The diagnosis of unexplained infertility can be even more confusing and extremely frustrating for people because it's unexplained!

This whole process can make you feel broken, confused, and angry. And then you feel ashamed for feeling angry or jealous when all your friends are having babies. Plus, everything is happening inside your body, so while the outside of your body looks fine, clearly it's not. There's a big disconnect. It becomes a very obsessive and heartbreaking experience.

♥ ♡ ♥

THE BIG SHIFT IN YOUR THINKING
By: Michelle

As women, we're often conditioned to believe our one sole purpose in life is to have children. All your life you're told, "Don't have sex or you'll get pregnant!" You go through your teen years believing sex is the magical road to pregnancy. So when you start trying and realize there's a lot more moving parts and pieces . . . Well, that's a lot to take in.

To go from believing unprotected sex leads to pregnancy to finding out your road to parenthood will look vastly different than what you learned in school is a huge shift—one that asks you to fundamentally change long-held beliefs about yourself and the world. It's not only a hard shift to make, but there's virtually no emotional support in the reproductive medical field to address that sudden transition. It's a very quick flip of your dream life. One minute you're fantasizing about your future nursery and the next a doctor is telling you you're infertile. It's like your life comes to a screeching halt in a single instant. Growing up, it felt like all the women in my life got pregnant easily and right away. My mom had three kids under three. So I never once imagined a life where getting pregnant would be a problem for me. What I naively didn't realize is that infertility isn't a "me" problem, it's a "we" problem.

My husband was the one who suspected something might be wrong, He casually mentioned it a couple of times. And since that wasn't what I wanted to hear I became a pro at brushing it off. "Oh, it's just taking a while . . . " or "We're not tracking it right . . . " or "We're not following my cycle . . . " You know, all the things you come up with so that you don't have to face the reality that something might be wrong. After five or six months of trying on our own, my husband took matters into his own hands by buying an over-the-counter test from the pharmacy, which, little did I know, came back funky. After getting the official semen analysis from the urologist, he broke the news to me by giving me the name and number of an RE to call: "It's time for you to get checked out too." I was simultaneously terrified and relieved. On the one hand, I didn't want to believe this was happening, and on the other, I was relieved to hopefully get some answers and expedite our baby-making process.

Growing up, I never felt like I fit in and when we got diagnosed with Male Factor Infertility it wasn't any different. Suddenly WE were part of the infertility community, but did I belong here!? I spent a lot of time grappling with what this all meant. For me. For our relationship. Was it ok and safe to seek out support in the infertility community if I technically didn't hold the diagnosis? If you've ever felt like you don't belong because your story is different, because you don't personally carry the diagnosis, because you already have a kid (or two or three), because you chose to do IVF for an entirely different reason . . . I just want to say I SEE YOU.

There are so many paths that lead to infertility and even to IVF. And while our stories may look different, at some point, each of us must grapple with the same shift of shedding an old identity and embracing a new one that involves infertility and IVF. So, no matter what led you here, no matter how or why you ended up on this hard road, let me offer you one more shift that will bring you comfort on the extra hard days: Your story is valid and you are not alone.

♥ ♡ ♥

THE LONELIEST PLACE IN THE WORLD
By: Keisha

As Black women, we are expected to pop babies out. You get married, or you don't get married, but you have babies. And that's just the way it is. I've been with my husband for twenty years, since we were sixteen, so the first thing after we got married was, "Why don't you have babies? What's wrong with you?" Even last week, his cousin was like, "Well, why don't you guys have a baby?" Why are you asking me what is wrong instead of educating yourself on the possibility that maybe we just don't want children or can't have them and it's not your business to ask? It's very painful when people are in your business about children when they have no idea and it all goes back to the thinking that we're just highly fertile as Black women.

My mom is one of nine. She had two miscarriages before me and my brother, but she has two children; her sister has four or five; all of her brothers and their wives have children; all of my cousins have children; some of my cousin's children have children. So I am the only one in our family that has a battle with infertility. So it's like the loneliest place in the world. Not a lot of other Black women have ever spoken about it, and we have been suffering in silence for so long. So I think it's important for people to say, "Hey, you know, I went through this battle and you're not by yourself, you're not the only person in the universe that fought through this, and it means a lot to talk about it."

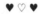

It was after our fourth transfer attempt that the RE suggested a myomectomy to remove the huge fibroid I had. We had spent several cycles trying to navigate around the huge fibroid that had found a way to nuzzle and embed itself into the perfect position where it made my transfers close to an hour. Do I need to mention how full my bladder felt as I tried my best to relax through it all? Listening to my carefully prepared playlist on my iPod and trying to ignore how much I wanted to pee. We wanted to try everything to avoid the huge surgery and several months of recovery that could set any IVF attempts back almost a year. My inability to carry my pregnancies past the first trimester after each successful transfer is what finally made the myomectomy unavoidable. I had to have the surgery.

Myomectomy is a big deal. It is a large abdominal incision, requires a few days in the hospital, and a long recovery period. Add to that the fear that the surgical removal of fibroids may affect the lining of the uterus and may make any future pregnancies harder. I had the surgery and it was a hard recovery. I had complications post-surgery and had a longer than expected hospital stay. My mother-in-law and my mother both flew out to California in the weeks afterward to help me get back on my feet. I was able to begin IVF again almost eight months later but was completely surprised to find out that nothing had changed. I was still getting pregnant and still having a miscarriage early in the first trimester. My frustration level was off the charts. How was this crap still happening? After everything I had been through, after everything my body had been through, how was the outcome not any different? First, it was the endometriosis, so that was a surgery. Then, it was the polyps, so they were removed. The fibroids were taken out—what was left? It was completely infuriating. There were no answers, there was no understanding. There was nothing that I felt could be fixed, since no one was able to determine what was wrong.

I remember being in a silent fury about the injustice of it all. I thought that if only I knew what was wrong, if only I knew the specific diagnosis for my infertility, I would be able to handle it. In my mind, it was the unexplained part of infertility that was the problem. I told myself that if only I had concrete answers, I would be able to move forward and I would not be angry. This was the thought that I carried with me for years. I thought this until I met a young woman in my support group who was only twenty-four. She had joined the group because at twenty she had been diagnosed with a condition that had rendered her infertile. You see, she knew exactly why she was infertile. She had solid and specific answers to all her questions. Knowing exactly what caused her infertility did nothing at all to lessen the pain and anguish she felt in her heart. It hit me that I wasn't mad that I didn't know why. I was mad and hurt because, whether you know why or not, it is always unfair.

Having a reason was not going to be a magic bullet to give me any clarity or greater insight or acceptance. Knowing why was not going to make me feel better. Being infertile was always going to hurt.

REFLECTION

"You Google infertility and you don't see me."

-Unknown

What hurts more than being invisible and marginal to the dominant conversation? For me, it was the shame of it all. The feeling of shame I had when diagnosed with infertility and undergoing treatment was one of the most toxic things in my life. It was also the hardest to shake. It made absolutely no sense either. Why was I feeling so much shame over something that I had no control over? Still, I carried the weight of my personal shame and the feeling of somehow being less than. Every day and every night, the little voice nagging in my head would ask, *What did I do to make this happen?* Shame and guilt exist together when you find yourself fighting back against your own body. Was I not meant to be a mother? Was my infertility part of a grand plan? Was I somehow being punished? So often, I felt bombarded by negative thoughts of my own making.

The voices from friends and family that were meant to be supportive oftentimes were quite the opposite. I couldn't count the times I was told to just relax. "It will happen in its own time. Go on vacation. Stop worrying about it. You work too hard. You need to lose weight. You need to put some meat on your bones. You need to change your diet. Try exercising. Try resting more. Did you try acupuncture? Did you try these herbs? Stop eating dairy. I know someone who was fifty and had a baby." On, and on, and on with the well-meaning advice that did more to make me scream internally and want to pull my hair out than it did to help in any way. This was how I quickly learned the difference between intention and impact. All the people who loved me intended to be supportive and helpful. The impact was that they reinforced and hammered in all my insecurities and the fact that I was indeed broken. I was also alone. This happened to everyone else, which felt especially true because the common thought is that Black and Brown women are supposed to be hyper-fertile. Didn't the messaging from the media shove the narrative down my throat that the problem Black women faced was that we were too fertile? We had too many babies, so how on earth do I wind up being the Black woman that can't have one?

This is the very reason why these hard conversations among women of color are necessary and why they need to impact the larger world. Women of color are not what's broken. The system that is supposed to support us is broken. Race is not the issue in infertility care and treatment. It is structural racism that is the problem in properly identifying our needs. Bias in the medical field plays a huge part in the timeliness of diagnosis and care. Knowing this bias exists makes it hard to fully trust the system. Feeling isolated within a system I didn't fully trust made me feel like a ghost, moving through every room yet not being seen or heard. I felt invisible in every stage of my journey because I was never able to see a mirror that reflected my struggle. Everything looked the same, yet none of it looked like me. It's impossible to claim space when we are not even allowed in the room.

So, let's talk about race. If you are reading this and you are not a woman of color, it can be easy to be dismissive or defensive around race. I am not speaking just around infertility, but racial implications around life in general. I totally get it. It is not comfortable to talk about race, and even less so to face our own implicit biases and blind spots. The facts are clear: racism exists and it affects and instructs the medical care and treatment of non-white women to their detriment. If you are white, none of the racial issues I am speaking about apply directly or individually to you. If your first reaction to racial discussions is to think "not me" or "not all white people," you are unintentionally centering yourself and your personal feelings into the conversation. Speaking openly about racial bias is not a way to target you or make you feel guilty. Centering your feelings of discomfort distracts from the real work we all have to do to dismantle structural racism. Sit in the discomfort, lean into the conversation. Changing your perspective and recentering the narrative—these things lead to greater inclusivity and true empathy. Keep focused on that.

It is structural and institutional racism that allow the experience and healthcare of women of color to be diminished. If you are white, you are part of the dominant social group; all standards are set up for you and measured against you. Any deviation from your norm is othered. Since white people have the vast majority and power in medical settings, they are in the position to only represent and consider their own perspective. Just imagine, if infertility sucks when you are white, it can be downright horrific if you are a woman of color. So, while the experiences of white women can be wildly different, whiteness is a central component of the specific experience that gets pushed to the forefront of the conversation. So, this is where we land. The racial divide exists and it affects women of color before we even step into the waiting room.

A 2016 University of Virginia[1] study found that the majority of white medical students believed in false biological differences, such as Black people having thicker skin, nerve endings that were not as sensitive, and were not as susceptible to pain as white people. These assumptions lead to real-world differences in diagnosis, treatment, and pain management for patients. This study formally acknowledges what non-white people have known and experienced all along. This is a major cause of distrust in the system. We know ahead of time that we may not be treated the same. We know our diagnosis and treatment will not be the same. Since the care is not the same, we know the outcome will be different and negatively affected.

If you need more proof, look no further that the Black maternal death rate in the United States. Black women are two and a half times more likely to die giving birth than other women.[2] These are deaths that are usually preventable and yet we're living in a moment when being Black and pregnant can also be a death sentence.

Black women have suffered medical injustice for centuries. Enslaved people were not even considered people. As far back at the 1800's there are documented writings from physicians that claim Black people do not experience any pain. The father of modern gynecology, Dr. J. Marion Sims was able to make breakthrough advances in the field because of the experimentation on non-consenting Black women without any anesthesia. This history is as ugly as it is painful, and it's a haunting legacy that lingers today in every medical interaction.

1   Kelly M. Hoffman et al, "Racial bias in pain assessment and treatment recommendations, and false beliefs about biological differences between blacks and whites," *Proceedings of the National Academy of Sciences of the United States of America (PNAS)*, 113, no. 16 (April 2016): https://doi.org/10.1073/pnas.1516047113

2   Elizabeth Chuck, "The U.S. finally has better maternal mortality data. Black mothers still fare the worst," *NBC News*, January 30, 2020. https://www.nbcnews.com/health/womens-health/u-s-finally-has-better-maternal-mortality-data-black-mothers-n1125896

That is the thing about implicit bias: it is quiet and subtle. What so many white people get wrong is in the thinking that racism overt and only bad people are racist. But I know that a very good person can unintentionally harbor a great deal of implicit bias. Ilana Ressler, MD writes, "Solely seeing IVF depicted as a white woman's experience can lead to doctors internalizing the stereotype, affecting referrals to reproductive specialists, medical research, and outreach to particular populations."[3] Society constantly upholds the messages that whiteness is central and all other experiences are the periphery. Women of color can find themselves in the position of trying to walk the tightrope of advocating for better care without falling into the "angry Black woman" stereotype. "We were never 'angry Black women,'" states Rachel Elizabeth Cargle in a social media post. "We were always reactive Black women. Reactive to the ways white America dismissed our bodies and silenced its voices and valued us as people only as it best fit their own white American needs. The history and realities they forgot in your text books and news headlines but forever a part of our reality."[4]

It is easy to be exasperated when no one in my world (before I was thirty-eight) ever really spoke to me about my fertility. I heard a lot about not getting pregnant. All the education in school was about preventing pregnancy and STD's. There was nothing about fertility, fertility issues, fibroids, endometriosis, PCOS, or polyps. I can't help but think how often the prevailing trope of the hyper-fertile Black woman came into play.

---

3   Ilana Ressler, "Dispelling Myths Surrounding Fertility and Women of Color," *Reproductive Medicine Associates of Connecticut,* July 13, 2020. https://www.rmact.com/fertility-blog/dispelling-myths-surrounding-fertility-and-women-of-color

4   Rachel Elizabeth Cargle (@rachel.cargle), "Saturday School: Confronting the History of Black Women and Forced Sterilization," Instagram, August 15, 2020. www.instagram.com/rachel.cargle

I was twenty-one and in college when I was finally diagnosed with endometriosis, more than a decade after I first told my doctor about my symptoms and pain. A decade during which I was brushed off and ignored when I cried every month. A time during which more than one doctor told me that my pain was not as bad as I said it was and that I needed to stop complaining. The only advice I received after my first surgery was to try and have babies as soon as possible. No one spoke to me about the serious implications of infertility and what that might mean. I never even knew there was an option or possibility of freezing my eggs. No one ever talked to me about fibroids—the fibroids that grew so large I was forced to have a radical hysterectomy at forty-six. I found out at thirty-five that fibroids not only run in my family, but that my mother and grandmother suffered from them as well. I never knew how devastating the presence of fibroids could be to my body. "Studies show that African-American women suffer fibroids 2 to 3 times more than white women," says McLeod OB/GYN Dr. Monica Ploetzke. "We also know that Black women tend to experience fibroids at a younger age and often more severely than their white counterparts."

Dr Ploetzke goes on to say, "One estimate is that 25% of African-American women will suffer from fibroids by the age of 25 and 80% will have them by age 50 (compared with 70% for white females). Because Black women suffer fibroids at an earlier age, they also are 2 to 3 times more likely to undergo surgery."[5] Why is this information not plastered in neon signs in every doctor's office or screamed during every mention of female health? If you

5   Monica Ploetzke, medical reviewer, "Fibroids: Greater in African-American Women than White. Why?" *McLeod Health* (blog), 2020. https://www.mcleodhealth.org/blog/fibroids-greater-in-african-american-women-than-white-but-why

are not given the pertinent information, you don't have the opportunity to make the right decisions.

BE OPEN

By: Lola

Being willing to share the journey and the process is important. Don't stay silent. I think bigger things like conception and fertility don't discriminate, we don't get it or not get it, just because we're one race the other. Your journey and your experience is valid. My experience is valid, and to be able to have a community and to have a sisterhood, and people who understand you and support you, that's huge, that makes the difference.

♥ ♡ ♥

What I am trying to get across is that acknowledging the history of racism and your privilege within its structures is not intended to make you feel guilty, it is intended to make you aware of the very issues we all have to fight to correct. Nothing will ever improve for us collectively as women unless we fight to do better by all women. Black maternal death rates exist because of financial obstacles, lack of access to health care, and disparities in prenatal treatment: all of that is tied to structural racism. These death rates are real-time indicators of the health of our entire nation. As women, we have to fight and do better for each other. That is the only way any of us will thrive and more forward.

Chapter Three

TREATMENT:
What Will it Take to Make a Baby?

*"IVF, taking the fun out of
procreation since 1978."*

-Unknown

I can't be the only one who thought that treatment was going to be easy. I look back and try to understand where all my misinformation came from. It is a double-edged sword. While it is amazing to be in a time where more women are speaking openly, there is a huge disconnect between the glossy magazine story and the reality that hits when the first big, very expensive box of meds arrives at your door from the fertility pharmacy. Laid out on the table in all its glory: pills, vials, patches, creams, needles (some of them looking unnecessarily huge), pens, alcohol swabs—it is all unnerving. Oh yeah, if you think that IVF always works the first time, get ready to be disappointed very quickly. Reproductive spaces that have utterly failed in being honest about what it means to go through infertility treatments. When you find out exactly what treatment entails, it is more than daunting, it is almost insurmountable. Money, class, or race don't make the daily reality any easier. Broadway star, Renee Elise Goldsberry of *Hamilton* fame openly lamented about the difficulty of infertility treatment in her 2016 Tony Award acceptance speech. She said, "I would just love to say that if you know anything about me you know I have spent the last ten years of my life but some would consider the life blood of a woman's career just trying to have children.

And I get to testify in front of all of you that the Lord gave me Benjamin and Brielle and he still gave me this."[1]

♥ ♡ ♥

IT CAN WRECK YOUR NERVES
By: Alicia

In the parenthood journey, every day brings a new concern. No time to worry about tomorrow. Do I have to take all of these medications? Is there an alternative to the PiO IM shot? Will the eggs survive thawing? Will they fertilize? Will they make it to day three? Will we have to transfer both? What if one does not survive freezing or thawing? What if something happens to both? Will that embryo make it to day five? Will we have a positive pregnancy test? Can I stay pregnant? Will this baby love me? Will others accept this baby as mine? *It can wreck your nerves!!* I wish I could say I immediately put all my cares on the altar, but I didn't. Sometimes it gets me down. Sometimes, especially lately, it is simply overwhelming. I have decision-making fatigue. I've done all I can do; I can't do anymore. I just wake up saying, "Lord, don't hand me a decision today. Take it away or make it super easy. I. Just. Can't." And I am okay with being honest with God. We don't have to wear a mask with God. Whew!

---

1   Melissa Willets, "Fertility Struggles and a Tony: Hamilton's Renee Elise Goldsberry Opens Up In Her Acceptance Speech," *Parents,* June 13, 2016. https://www.parents.com/pregnancy/everything-pregnancy/fertility-struggles-and-a-tony-hamiltons-renee-elise-goldsberry-opens

My first attempt at an IVF cycle was a total bust. The birth control pills and Lupron depressed my system too much and no amount of stimming would make my eggs grow. The next try ended with a fizzle and not a bang. It failed horribly when my one bitchy alpha egg grew so large that it refused to allow any other eggs to grow. Close to thirty days of stimulation drugs and all I had to show was one egg. My doctor admitted defeat and sent me home. That day, canceling my cycle felt more like a get-out-of-jail-free card than a disappointment. I left the doctor's office, called my friend Katie to meet me for brunch, and then proceeded to overindulge in all the delicacies that IVF had forbidden: mimosas, Bloody Marys, wine, coffee, chocolate soufflé. Anything and everything that was denied to me during my quest to be perfect for my transfer now made its way to the table. Katie cheered and cried with me in equal measure; she was there to celebrate and commiserate with me. After a failed cycle, we all need a bit of Katie in our lives. Someone who joins us at the table with no judgment, just understanding, love, and unconditional support.

♥ ♡ ♥

IT FEELS NEVER-ENDING
By: Keisha

This is a long, frustrating story. We got married at twenty-four. At around twenty-five, we said, "Let's try to have a baby." But nothing was happening. I had always had pain and heavy bleeding with my periods, so when I went to the doctor and they said, "Well, you have two cysts on both ovaries, so that means when you get pregnant, you're going to have twins," I thought, *Oh, this is fantastic, this is great. Who wouldn't want to have two babies at once?* A couple of years passed and we started going to fertility specialists. We did three IUIs and nothing. We did all the testing. Nothing. "You're perfectly healthy," I was told. "We don't know why you're not getting pregnant."

So we stopped for a while, and when I was about twenty-nine or thirty, we went back to it. They did the HSG where they put the dye in—they did everything. They could not find any issues. We went through the IVF cycle; they retrieved thirteen eggs and inseminated them with my husband's semen. The day that we were supposed to go in and do the transfer, my doctor told us that after twelve had fertilized, all of the embryo's were gone. All of them had expired. We had no idea why, but they couldn't do our transfer. I saw the doctor a month later and she said, "Well, we don't know what's going on, we don't know what happened, and my advice to you is to lose weight, save money on Girl Scout cookies, and come see me again in a couple of years when you have enough money." I would never see that doctor again because her bedside manner was horrible—she was horrible.

A couple of years passed and I was still having all this pain. I went to my gynecologist and she says, "There is no kind of gynecological issue, go have a colonoscopy." What? Yeah, that was my face. So, I got the colonoscopy thinking that my doctor knows what she's doing—I trusted her and that's what I did. There was no problem with my colonoscopy results.

Finally, I began going to the doctor that I'm currently seeing. I was thirty-four at the time. She found that I have PCOS, fibroids, and polyps, so she went in to remove them. We did another cycle of IVF, and she thought that my ovarian reserve was low, so now we needed an embryo donor or an egg donor. Our hearts were broken. We said, "We can't have a biological child, but let's do this, let's move forward." My uncle who we were very close to, who was also our pastor, ended up linking us up with someone who happened to have been through IVF and had an embryo leftover that they wanted to donate. Amazing! He connected us with her and the next day, after he gave her my phone number, my uncle passed away. He kind of put his hand into it and then he passed away, so we started going through all the legal stuff and getting everything ready. The day after Mother's Day, the donor said, "I changed my mind, we don't want to do this now."

So again, our hearts were absolutely crushed. Where do we go now at this point? My cousin, who was my uncle's daughter, and I want to continue his legacy, so she decided to donate her eggs to me. We are currently in the process of going through that, she's stimulation drugs as we speak, so hopefully, God willing this will work out.

I found out quickly after two dismal attempts using my own eggs that we would need to use an egg donor. No matter how long I stimmed, my eggs were completely unresponsive. I never did a successful transfer with my own egg. I never even made it to retrieval day. It was a hard thing to hear from the doctor. My eggs, my DNA, my biological connection—none of that was going to be a part of the baby equation anymore. I didn't know how to feel. I left the office emotionally numb. How do I even start to find the egg donor for the child I would carry, deliver, and be a mother to in every way? Would I feel different carrying a child that wasn't biologically mine? Would my husband feel different? Does he think I am less of a woman? He very quickly put me at ease by telling me it was all going to be ok. "Look," he said, "if you needed a lung, we would find you a lung. You need an egg, we're getting you an egg." And that is how we began the great egg hunt.

It definitely would have been infinitely easier to be white and looking for a donor. Every site we found on the internet for Egg Donor agencies had hundreds, if not thousands of smiling, beautiful white donors. I was lucky to find an agency that had seven Black donors. In the end, I was so frustrated at how hard it was to find a Black egg donor, I slammed down the computer screen and yelled out loud, "Brown! She just needs to be any kind of Brown!" And there is no guidebook for how to choose a donor. Do you look for the prettiest, the healthiest, the smartest? Do you choose the young woman who wrote the best essay? Do you look for the person who you would want to adopt and add to your family? If you know or have a relationship with the donor, I would imagine that you would have a whole other set of questions. We went with someone who most matched me physically, even though that someone ended up being half-Black and half-Filipino. We never met her, on the advice of the agency, but we had a ton of pictures of her and wrote her a letter. I started the letter by telling her that even though we would never meet, I loved her and would love her forever for her incredible gift, that she was always going to live in our hearts, and that we were going to be grateful to her for the rest of our lives. She put herself through all the nastiness and shots of stimming and was able to give us over fifteen eggs of excellent quality from her retrieval.

We were finally ready to do IVF using donor eggs and were ready and excited for a fresh cycle. Tommaso was going to leave a sperm sample during the egg donor's retrieval. I love my husband dearly, but, honestly, that day, I wanted to throw him out of a window. He came out of the small side donor room by the nurses' station holding his cup of liquid gold with an extremely pissed-off look on his face. I was worried. What on earth could have happened in that room to make him angry? I thought between the two of us, he definitely had the easier and way more pleasurable task that day. What was he going to do that he had not done thousands of times before? I was so concerned and wanted to console him until he told me what he was mad about: He wasn't worried about me or wondering if we would have success with the egg donor. Nothing had gone "wrong" and he wasn't upset about the cost of yet another procedure. He was mad because he didn't like the selection of reading materials and videos that were provided in the room. That's right, his complaint that day was about the porn. My biggest cheerleader, my biggest support, the one who carried me through all the horrific things that came with infertility was upset because he didn't like the porn. He didn't like any of the magazines or movies (nothing featured women of color) and he said he couldn't get comfortable because he didn't want to sit down or touch anything in the room. I tried—I really and truly tried—to stay calm. I wanted to find a way to be empathetic, but I exploded. You can blame it on the hormones, but honestly, I was pissed on principle. I had been through surgery, had been a human pin cushion—sticking myself multiple times a day with needles, had changed my whole life to try to get pregnant, and this man was going to look me in the face and say he didn't like the porn?! I lost it. It wasn't our best moment as a couple. I was exhausted with everything I had been through, mentally and physically, and was not prepared to have Tommaso walk out of a room after masturbating and complain about not liking the pictures. Are you kidding me? Hell. No. I imagine that he is still recovering from me telling him off. I mean, who cares about the porn? We are trying to make a baby the only way we can, so you pull it together, get in the room, do what has to be done, and do not ever talk to me about how you don't like the nudie magazines EVER again! That was the first and last time he ever opened his mouth again about sperm samples. Now, I can say that this story is one of our favorite IVF memories and the one that makes us laugh the hardest. It is true what they say about comedy, it really does come from tragedy over time.

♥ ♡ ♥

THE STRUGGLE IS REAL

By: Jenelle

My husband and I got married in 2016, he had just finished his Ph.D., and I was just finishing up my first year in grad school. I was excited to get married and we've always wanted children, but it wasn't the right time since I wanted to finish school and get a good job. It was always in the back of my mind. We kind of set a rough timeline: 2018 was going to be the year. I was looking forward to it because it was what I wanted ever since I was a little girl. Finally, in December of 2017, I had secured a job in my field and was in my last semester of grad school, and was feeling good about the future—I started the baby fund. I was starting to take prenatal vitamins and reading all the books. My husband is a bit older and I had heard that sometimes when the partner is older, it can take longer; I'm a planner, so when it came time, I wanted to know exactly what I needed to do to make this happen as quickly as possible. I was realistic. I was so excited to finally start our family, but in the back of my mind, I knew it could take longer. My brother had to go through IVF with his wife. My husband's sister got married late, so it took her and her husband three years and major dietary changes to conceive. With all that background, we acknowledged that while my husband is in good health, you just never know.

So, I think that's why six months before we started trying, I was doing all my research and my prep. I bought a fertility tracker bracelet that took my temperature at night and I was using ovulation strips and everything. We even planned a European cruise for our anniversary. I was going to try all the wine in Europe and then I was going to come back and we were going to make babies. That was the plan.

We started trying. Nothing the first month. I wasn't worried. They said it doesn't always happen the first month; I was fine. Then the second month went by, and then the third, and the fourth, so I thought, *Okay, hold up now, I know we're doing this right. We're getting the timing right. What is happening here?*

I didn't have the patience that some people have about all of this. Some people wait the full six months, but by cycle four, I was talking to my doctor. She ordered blood tests for me and a sperm analysis for my husband. We got the results back and there was no sperm found in his sample. That was devastating because I didn't even know that was possible. There are supposed to be millions in there, and there's not a single one? So then the doctor said, "You need to work with the urologist. I'm going to refer you to an infertility center as well."

My husband already had a urologist from when he had kidney stones a few years back, so we started out with him, but then I didn't think infertility was really his thing, so we found a different urologist in the same practice who was a little bit more well-versed in male-factor infertility. We started doing some testing there, and repeat sperm analyses showed the same thing. Still, his hormone levels looked great and his blood work was normal, so they weren't finding anything that could have been the cause of his abnormal sample. We developed a plan with the urologist to do a testicular biopsy to see if they could get the harvest that way, and then we were working along with the IVF center, getting the rest of my testing out of the way, just so that if they were able to harvest from him, we could jump right into IVF.

So even though the IVF consultation was in March of 2019, my husband's biopsy wasn't scheduled until June, which meant there was just a lot of "hurry up and wait." In the meantime, I got all my testing done, and I was still saving in the baby fund and trying to be optimistic. Finally, it was time for his surgery and it was also his birthday. I know it was the worst birthday ever. He was recovering in our room when we got the call that unfortunately, there was no sperm found in the testicular biopsy. Part of the biopsy was used to potentially harvest the sperm, and then the other part was used to diagnose what was going on. We were able to learn that he had a genetic condition where he doesn't have the parts to make a mature sperm cell. This condition was so rare—why was this happening to us?

It was a tough blow. I think for him it was hard to even come to terms with the fact that it was "on him" that we couldn't have a baby and he felt the crush of "I'm letting my wife down and I'm less of a man." None of that was true but it was really rough. Those few months were the lowest point in our marriage because he had all these feelings going on. I wasn't blaming him and I wasn't looking at him differently—I was trying to be very supportive—but I felt like I didn't know how to be supportive or how to help him feel better. I told him, "At the end of the day, I want to have a family with you, and there are ways that we can still make that happen." I think he had a hard time getting past the initial shock and grief, and so we weren't quite on the same page, which I totally understood. I imagine if the roles were reversed, I probably would have needed more time to process things, so I gave time and space. I went to counseling because I felt like I needed to talk to someone and it was nice to have my feelings validated and to be better prepared to approach those conversations with him. It took a lot in those months to relearn how to talk to each other and be honest about what we wanted with each other. The truth for me was that I really couldn't imagine a life without having children, it's just something I always envisioned and wanted.

I loved my family dynamics growing up, and I wanted to recreate that. It's purely selfish, but that's what I wanted for my life, and so I think I made it clear to my husband that this is kind of a non-negotiable thing, and I still want to do this thing with you, maybe be open to other alternatives. I think in time, he was able to work through his own feelings and process that I was not looking at him like a failure or less of a man. I wasn't blaming him. I think that helped him to come around. Donor sperm was kind of our easy fix, so to speak, because it would still allow me to carry our children and we could still build our family—I could still have the pregnancy experience. We were going to have our family.

We started looking for donors. First, we were going to ask my husband's cousin because, for one, I just love this cousin—he's a great guy, and two, they look alike. Well, we found out that he had been secretly fighting a successful battle against testicular cancer that destroyed all his reproductive capabilities. The option for a known donor went right out the window. So we started looking at some different cryobanks and we made a bunch of accounts and came up with our list of criteria and what was important to us. It was harder than we thought to find someone that matched my husband's physical characteristics.

There was just the one that stood out and we thought, this is probably the closest we're going to get. But then the right one popped up one day. I said, "Look at this guy, he's got the hair, his face shape is similar, he's got your nose, like, this is great." The eyes were different but everything else was wonderful; they were similar in height and build, and it just fit. It felt meant to be when we found him. We certainly slept on it a little bit, but within the week, we were ready to pull the trigger.

We dove into IVF then. And honestly, I used to be afraid of needles and getting my blood drawn, so it was kind of funny to be doing these daily injections, and then up to three a day when I was doing stims. But I just kept thinking, *I'm doing this for our family, and I'm going to have everything I want on the other side of this.* I no longer have a needle phobia—that's one way to get over that fear, right?

♥ ♡ ♥

THE RED DRESS
By: Tasha and Kelli

Tasha: I know there is not a wrong way to do any of this, but we had no clue at all about what we were doing. We're two women, it was not going to just happen. Major plans had to be made and put in place. When we found a donor, we decided that we were just going to buy all the sperm, every canister, not just one or two, all of it. Then we called a specialist, one that we had never even seen before, and asked if we could ship it to their office for them to freeze. We weren't even patients yet. We called and asked, "Can you freeze our stuff, we'll pay for it?" They said yes and then we made our first appointment.

Kelli: Then I remember I was getting up early, getting dressed for our appointment day. I had been checking my own ovulation numbers, but that was all we were doing. We were not prepared for an IUI. We thought we could just walk into the office that day and say, "Ok, let's get this done." I am being serious.

We showed up for our appointment, and I have to talk about my outfit. It's funny to think about it now. I was dressed up. I was wearing a really cute red dress and had huge wedge heels on. We were dressed, we were ready, we were going to come in, get pregnant, and stroll out. The doctor came out and met us at the front desk. He stopped us in our tracks and took us back into his office. He told us, "I can take your money right now and you can do this today, or we can start at the beginning so you can do this the right way." So, that's when the process began. Still, I looked really great in my red dress.

Tasha: Yeah, you did.

I'm sure we could all join together and write another book around our Clomid stories alone. My personal kryptonite was Lupron and that horrible, terrible, no good progesterone-in-oil shot. I had already been unfortunate enough to suffer through months of Lupron shots in my early twenties. I was prescribed Lupron post-surgery to help combat my endometriosis. There was nothing like going through faux menopause and living through hot flashes at your sorority formal. My college boyfriend's mom even had to give me my Lupron shots one summer while I was visiting his family. She may not remember the names of all of her son's girlfriends, but I am fairly sure that all these decades later, after shooting Lupron into my butt, she definitely remembers mine.

I don't think I ever got "used" to all the shots, but I was forced to learn to live with them. It was the crazy schedule that almost broke me. I was legitimately terrified every day that I would take the wrong meds at the wrong time and completely mess up my entire cycle. My daily calendar was a color-coded, time-stamped fertility bible that I followed with fanatical devotion, without question. I took my needles and meds everywhere with me. I became adept at leaving work meetings, parties, dinners, and movies to dash to the bathroom and shoot up. I even pulled my car over for a quick fix of Menopur in a gas station bathroom. Not my finest moment, but it didn't matter where or when, if the schedule said it was time for a shot, I was going to take the shot. My poor stomach was a pin cushion littered with tiny black and blue bruises, looking like I had been attacked by hundreds of really angry infertility mosquitoes. Even today, just the smell of rubbing alcohol takes me right back to the tiny sting of those needles in my stomach.

When it came time for that huge progesterone-in-oil shot, I thought that this would be a great opportunity for my sweet husband to get involved and help out. I very quickly found out that our marriage vows (while covering promises to love, honor, and cherish) did not cover sticking a long, thick needle in your wife's butt. Tommaso just froze. I found out very late in the game that he had a huge fear of needles. Even though he wanted to be the most amazing husband, he was terrified that giving me the shot was going to hurt. Well, spoiler alert, the big shot did hurt but Tommaso struggled to help.

Our first attempt did not go well. I ended up shoving him away in absolute frustration and jabbing myself. I spent the rest of the night nursing my sore rear end with ice and heat. It took another two days before I realized that I was only going to be able to reach the same spot on my backside—the one that was already sore—before I told Tommaso he had to suck it up and help. We had to share the shot burden. So, we cobbled together a plan so Tommaso could get the job done. He would find an unbruised location and do the initial jab. He would then guide my hand so I could inject the progesterone and then I would pull out the needle. I also discovered that icing the area before the shot and sitting on a heated compress after the shot helped. It still hurt, but I was managing the pain and discomfort. Like practically everything about infertility treatments, the shots sucked!

I WAS SO USED TO THINGS NOT WORKING

By: Rhondette

I will start from the place that I remember starting, which is when I got married at forty-two. I didn't know if I would be able to have children because I was getting married so late, and I had never been pregnant before or tried to get pregnant before. My husband and I pretty much started trying to get pregnant the day that we got married and I did get pregnant in October of that year. Then I had my first miscarriage—that was really hard. I knew that people had miscarriages, but I didn't think I would have one. I don't remember exactly when I started going to a specialist, a reproductive endocrinologist, but after the miscarriage, I was thinking, *Well, if there's anything I could do . . . I don't know why the miscarriage happened, but if there's anything that I could do differently, I need to do differently. I'd like to know.* I talked to some friends who had also been in my doctor's care and was surprised to discover something like a secret society, the one you don't know you're in until you start talking to people and then women will tell you, "Oh, when I lost my first child," or, "I had a miscarriage in between children." That type of thing.

I went to two different clinics. The first one suggested IUI; we tried that a couple of times and we were not successful, so I switched to another specialist. The next endocrinologist found fibroids; I had my first fibroid surgery, which was awful, but I was still hopeful because I thought, *Okay, maybe that's the problem, I had a lot of fibroids.*

Two years had passed and then there was a recommendation about trying with an egg other than mine. We didn't start with donor eggs, but that was the initial recommendation when I went to the first reproductive endocrinologist. I was told, "Oh, we don't even want to try your eggs right away—donor egg only." Right there, that was the first recommendation, and I was thinking, *Well, wow, I haven't even really . . . that seems like a bit much.* I hadn't even heard of that possibility, so I didn't even know what she was talking about. Really? No one took any time to explain egg donation and the implications to me. So, long story short, I've been pregnant three times, but the second time was, again, naturally. We also tried a donor egg, and it didn't work; so we were going to try again. But by this time, another year had passed, and my fibroids had returned, so I had to have a second surgery, so this brings me up to April of 2017. By then, I had three pregnancies that were not successful, I'd had two surgeries and two IUI's, not necessarily in that order, but over the course of five years.

At this point, I told my husband that I felt like I was losing it emotionally, I just didn't know if I could keep getting all this disappointment. I asked him, "Well, what do you think about adoption?" He was fine with it, he said, "If you want to do it, I want to do it." I also joined a support group somewhere in the process, and that was helpful because I met five other ladies who were also dealing with trying to get pregnant (and stay pregnant) after having had several miscarriages. We are friends to this day.

I started talking on the phone to a friend of mine who had just adopted her second child. She was really honest about the process so I knew that if we decided to do this, it still could take a while, but we were ready to move forward. I was home from that second surgery and my friend had come to help. I asked if she would drive me to FedEx; the adoption agency told us there was a birth mom that requested our portfolio. I didn't talk about it because I think we had already done it about five times and nothing had happened. So I didn't want to even tell my friend that much, just that I was sending it off to the agency. About a week later, I got a call and the agency said that we had been selected, and I didn't believe it at first. She had to keep repeating it. She told us the birth mom liked our portfolio and we were the chosen ones! But I was so used to things not working, so used to hitting a wall, so used to disappointment, that it didn't quite connect. I always answered the phone expecting something negative, and that's sad to say, but it was just kind of a reflection after five years of disappointment.

We were told that the birth mom said she hadn't had any prenatal care, she was in denial for a long time. We didn't know the gender. She thought that she might have an abortion, but she had waited too long and decided on adoption. I said, "Well, do you think she's going to go through with it?" Again, I was expecting disappointment. The agency said "You know, I do. The fact that she came at this stage makes me think that she is really, really serious about doing this. I would like for you guys to meet and have a chance to just connect." I hung up the phone and I thought, *Okay, it seems like this might be happening.* But they also always tell you it's not final until it's final. I didn't create a registry, I didn't build a nursery.

I went back to work after taking time off to recover from surgery. It was a Tuesday in May. I told my boss that in June, I might have to go out on maternity leave. My job was extremely supportive. So the next day, Wednesday, I was sitting at my desk and the phone rings. I answered and heard "Hello, good morning, I just wanted to say congratulations. Your son was born this morning at 3:17 a.m."

To this day, I am still blown away by how it happened, because we hadn't met the birth mom. We hadn't done any of that stuff. I was waiting for the call to figure out the details, and now he was here. He was premature by eight weeks, so he was in the NICU. He was very sick when he was born, his lungs were not fully developed for the first week of life. When we got there, we met the birth mom. She was really nice. I met her mother, her sister, and two of her sister's kids. All of this and we still couldn't believe that she chose us. I told her that there wasn't anything I could say to express how deeply, deeply thankful I was for choosing me, for choosing us.

So, I have nothing but gratitude for her because if not for her, I wouldn't be a mom. She was thirty years old. She didn't have a lot of resources, had two other children, and she had lost her job. She had to move back in with her mom. The birth father was not a factor.

I wrote her a letter that I hoped she would read whenever she had second thoughts about her decision, and I gave her a beautiful watch and I wrote, "I just want you to know, every time you look at this watch, just remember that there will never be a time that he will not be loved and cherished." When we met, I hugged her. We hugged each other and I feel like that was the best scenario there could have been. You know, I don't know how those things normally happen, but I feel like God's grace manifested itself in that moment, and hopefully, she felt more comforted by that. After that, in separate rooms, we signed the papers and then someone said "Congratulations, Mom and Dad." I had never been called mom before; at that moment, life was beautiful. It was a surreal kind of moment, like somebody flipped a switch, because now we were in charge. We were in charge of his care, we were in charge of decisions—we were parents.

Have you noticed that when almost anyone who doesn't understand infertility finds out what you are going through, they are almost always incredulous? I know how I stared in amazement when my box of meds arrived from the fertility pharmacy, thinking to myself, *Wow, it's going to take all of this?* The people who don't know are always taken aback by what you are willing to endure physically to have a child. They always say some version of "Wow, I could never do that," or "Ew, I hate needles and shots." I came up with a reply. I say, "Look at your kid, if I told you that all you would have to do to have your child is to give yourself multiple shots several times a day, you would do it. You would do it without question and without hesitation. As a matter of fact, there is nothing you wouldn't do and no stone you would leave unturned if you thought that at the end of it all you would have your child."

REFLECTION

"You realize that a lot of it is luck, and you can't blame things on yourself."

-Chrissy Teigen

Say this loud and say this often because it can be easy to forget while you are in the middle of all of this, or when you're at the end of your journey. When blame consumes you and it is all that you can think about, day in and day out, try to remember this: your infertility, everything you are going through, it is all just one aspect of you. You are so much more. You are enough.

You are not broken. In fact, you are perfect and beautiful and amazing just the way you are!

Chapter Four

PREGNANCY & PREGNANCY AFTER INFERTILITY:
What Can I Expect Now That I am Expecting?

"If you conceived your child in fewer than six months, without the assistance of OPK's, without paying attention to your FP's and LP's and worrying about your FSH levels (or you don't know what these acronyms mean), then you have not TRIED to get pregnant. Pregnancy happened to you."

-Unknown

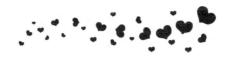

It finally happens, somehow, someway all the stars align and you see the two magical lines on the stick. One may be really faint, so you take a picture and ask your Facebook group what they think, but in your heart, you are starting to believe that it worked and you are pregnant. You don't want to hope, but you can't stop yourself. After everything you have been through, more than anything else at that moment you just want to believe. Even before the official blood test in the doctor's office, you just want to sit in the possibility and the magic that you are pregnant. Or maybe that was just me.

Of course, you have to sit through that horrific two-week wait. Is there a more perfect storm of anxiety and hope? You have been through the transfer and whether it was a fresh or frozen cycle, you lay there trying to relax with a full bladder while seeing that tiny embryo being put snugly inside of you. *Just stick, just stay, just let this work*, you may have silently prayed. You have a tiny hope that you try to contain—you could be pregnant. On the other hand, you seem to have all the time in the world to sit and think about how it may not have worked at all. I know that I can't be the only one that was taking daily pregnancy tests on the sly and examining the stick every day, holding it up in the light and searching for the faintest line.

There was something so perfect about that first transfer. I just knew it had worked. I don't know how, but I knew that the embryo had sticky vibes and I was pregnant. That first two-week wait was excruciating (honestly, no matter how many times you go through the 2 week wait, never gets any better). I peed on a stick every day for six days. I went through two boxes of pregnancy tests and each day the second line got darker and darker. I floated on air into the doctor's office for the blood test. I was wearing maternity clothes as soon as the results of the blood test came back positive. My numbers were awesome, more than doubling by the second blood test. When the nausea hit, I actually celebrated. Every single nasty side effect of being pregnant, I absolutely loved. It reminded me that I had succeeded. I won. I made infertility suck it! The IVF worked and that tiny embryo had attached. Baby Trinchieri was growing inside of me. I was going to be a mommy; I started plotting the full life of the child I was going to have. I had girl names and boy names all picked out, I was mentally decorating the nursery, and I admit to buying a ton of really cute onesies I saw at Target. I was pregnant, one of the lucky ones. I don't know if I will ever have such a pure sense of joy again.

FINDING THE JOY
THROUGH THE FEAR

By: Michelle, Infertility Coach and Infertility Patient

Here's what happens when you finally get pregnant on this journey, and it's not what you might be expecting. In fact, it's the opposite. When you get pregnant after this long, hard road, all of your previous patterns and bullshit come flooding back to you. I've seen it time and again with my clients; anytime we have a shift in our identity, anytime a new thing happens in our life, our brain goes into overdrive trying to process that new thing. This is so *normal* but can throw you for a complete loop. This is also why it's so important to *know* what these patterns and stories are, so you can shut them down and actually *enjoy* the thing you've worked so hard for. Don't let the trauma of this journey steal your joy. Don't let your brain trick you into thinking this too has to suck, because it doesn't.

So, how can you get back to center so you can find joy in this moment you've wished for for so long? You make sure you have tools in your belt to get you back to your grounded foundation. It might not happen in a day, but slowly, with tiny intentional steps each day, you'll get there. Here's my question for you: Do you know which way is North and how confident do you feel getting there? So that when your day comes, you can enjoy the crap out of your pregnancy rather than let the fear demons get in your way.

♥ ♡ ♥

GETTING PREGNANT DURING A GLOBAL PANDEMIC

By: Jenelle

It was time for our egg retrieval. I ended up with twenty-eight eggs retrieved and, ultimately, we had twelve high-graded embryos, which was great. Still, even before we went into the retrieval, our doctor reminded us that even though we had planned on a fresh transfer, my estrogen was through the roof and the fresh transfer would be ideal; so, we decided to freeze everything and do a frozen transfer in March.

At first, I was crushed and after the retrieval, I had a rough recovery; I developed Ovarian Hyper-Stimulation Syndrome (OHSS),[1] which can be a common response to the overstimulation of ovaries due to excessive hormones taken before egg retrieval. The ovaries swell and become extremely painful. I had a mild case, but it made my recovery very rough due to the pain and discomfort. I needed way more time off work than anticipated. I didn't feel so hot and I looked pregnant. I was in so much pain. Oh my gosh, there was so much pressure in my pelvis. I was not in any shape for a fresh transfer, so I accepted that our plans had changed to a frozen transfer in March.

We started all over in February with birth control and injections. When March rolled around, we did the baseline scan and started the estrogen pills. Then, just before I was supposed to start progesterone for the transfer, COVID-19 hit; they canceled our transfer a week before, and we were gutted. I was so upset because we had been through so much and then like that, it was over.

The clinic was canceling all procedures until further notice. They suggested going back on birth control and waiting until they re-open. They promised to get us back in as soon as they could. Birth control pills make me crazy; I didn't want to be on them indefinitely. It was a rough

---

1 "Ovarian Hyperstimulation Syndrome (OHSS) Fact Sheet," *The Patient Education Website of the American Society of Reproductive Medicine,* Revised 2014.   https://www.reproductivefacts.org/news-and-publications/patient-fact-sheets-and-booklets/documents/fact-sheets-and-info-booklets/ovarian-hyperstimulation-syndrome-ohss

time because I was transitioning now to working from home and navigating life in this uncharted territory of a health crisis. Emotionally, I felt like my dreams were shattered. I felt like we were so close to the finish line and then it was moved back again. I really tried to make the most of things, but I think not being able to live my regular life and get out—to do my fitness classes, go to brunch with my friends, go on dinner dates and things like that—I think it drained me even further. I didn't have my usual self-care routines to fall back on anymore.

Spring of 2020 was rough because of the pandemic, but once May came around, I got word that our IVF center was resuming procedures. I didn't know how to feel. There was still a pandemic going on and who knew when it was going to be over? Do we feel safe pursuing treatment and potentially getting pregnant now? After agonizing over it for a couple of weeks, I think we came to the conclusion that neither one of us was getting any younger, especially my husband. He was already getting a late start at fatherhood, and then with all these delays thrown on top, not knowing if or when this virus was going away, we thought, *can we wait indefinitely?* After weighing all the pros and cons and being realistic about what we could do to keep ourselves safe, we felt comfortable calling and seeing when the IVF center could get us in. We were able to schedule a transfer for June 23rd, but I couldn't even get excited; I felt like this was "take three." We were supposed to have our transfer in January—that got canceled. We were supposed to have our make-up transfer in March—that got canceled. You couldn't tell me that this one wasn't going to get canceled either, so I didn't let myself get excited. The IVF center kept trying to reassure me like, "Listen, we have a better sense of the COVID situation now, we don't anticipate shutting down again." It was probably the day I had to start the progesterone that I thought, *Okay, we're really doing this.*

I started to get excited and let myself feel like, *This is real, we're finally having our chance.* Sure enough, transfer day rolls around, and it was a super quick process; we got our picture of the embryo and we were on our way.

Wow, we actually did it. It was so weird, but it became real in those moments, and from there, it was a waiting game. I did my best to keep myself occupied and eating well and taking walks outside because I wasn't going anywhere. I'd been working from home full-time and Paul had taken over the grocery shopping for me so that I could minimize my exposure to anything dangerous. I didn't have any pregnancy symptoms.

I wondered if the transfer worked; I didn't feel different. But then, seven nights after the transfer, I just . . . I was thinking about a happy memory, right, the day we met our dog and we knew we wanted to adopt her—it was love at first sight and I had to have her. I started sobbing. Under normal circumstances, I'm not a crier, but it was uncontrollable for a good ten minutes straight, and my husband was looking at me like, "What is wrong with you? Are you okay? What happened? We were just talking about a happy thing. Why are you crying?" So, I took that as a sign that maybe the transfer had worked, because that was not me.

The next morning, I snuck around and took some tests, wanting to try to surprise my husband. Sure enough, I got some blazing positive results. Two years after we started trying, it worked. I had accumulated some baby things over the years—little booties, onesies, and storybooks—so I put together a small gift box with a few of those things in it. Then I put the positive tests in with them, including a digital one that said "Pregnant." I felt like a guy needs to see it spelled out. I didn't want any questions. It was for real.

My husband's birthday was a week before, so I said, "Oh, hey, honey, some of your presents were a little late in the mail. I have them here for you." I hit my phone and started recording. He opened the box and everything was buried in wrinkled confetti. First, he pulled out booties and was like, "Oh, these are cute," and then the next thing he pulled out was the little baggy with the tests and he said, "You're pregnant." He came and gave me a big bear hug and it was adorable. Fortunately, that transfer worked and I am at the thirteen-week mark tomorrow.

I'm feeling good and we are happy, but even in the beginning of the pregnancy, we had some scares. You get that positive test on the stick and it's amazing, but the actual blood test doesn't come until a full two weeks after the transfer. In my first test, my levels were super high. Then, I repeated the test two days later, and the numbers hadn't doubled— they had only risen by half, which made everyone worried. My head was spinning. *Oh my god, no, please don't tell me something's wrong.* Had this little thing planted in the wrong place? I had to go in to the clinic the next day; waiting until the next morning was torture and I was a mess. I was crying in bed, I was so upset. We started googling and we read that something could be wrong. We went in for our ultrasound, and there it was. The doctors saw the gestational sac and the yolk sac. I was five weeks and everything was right where it was supposed to be. "So, this is good, right? This is what we want to see at five weeks?" The nurse said, "Yes, let's be cautiously optimistic."

What does that even mean? I was celebrating that it wasn't in one of my tubes. This comment came from a nurse practitioner who I hadn't seen much of and we were a little put-off by her demeanor. Now, I had been doing my own research and it seemed that once your HCG (Human Chorionic Gonadotropinthe, the pregnancy hormone) gets to a certain point, it takes longer to double, so if you're rolling in with a really high number already, it may just need to increase and not double. The staff weren't acknowledging that at all.

The next week we went in and we saw the fetal pole and we heard the heartbeat, and it was perfect. It was great. The embryo was growing.

At around six weeks and three days I had awful cramping, followed by some brown spotting when I woke up. I was getting ready for work and I was terrified that something bad was happening. I was devastated and scared so I called the doctor and told them I needed an ultrasound and that I was very worried. They scheduled me immediately. By the time my appointment rolled around, I had pretty much figured out that the awful cramping was gas, but the pain had been in the general vicinity of where the uterus was—it was really low. I didn't know if it was my uterus or not and with the spotting, I was still concerned. Fortunately, the baby had grown and its heartbeat was great; they thought that maybe my cervix was just a little bit irritated. Being pregnant was one scare after the next, every little thing is heightened so much. It felt like every week there was something new. At our next appointment, we had another nurse practitioner and she didn't know how to use the vaginal ultrasound machine. With every other person, they put it in and the picture was clear on the screen—you look and there's the baby. I don't know what she was doing, but we were looking at my intestines. "That doesn't even look like my uterus," I said. It was awful. We would get a little glimpse of the baby and then it would be gone and she was saying, "Oh, it's hiding." Eventually, she got the clearest image that she could get, and she told us that the baby was measuring small. Then she said, "Oh, the heartbeat is a little bit slower than last week." So, I started freaking out again that something was happening to the baby. I panicked, I froze, I couldn't even think because it sounded like she was telling me this was not a viable pregnancy. Thankfully, my husband was there. He spoke up and said it didn't seem right and asked if there was a doctor available to take a look. I was so glad he asked because our doctor did come down and did another ultrasound; we saw the baby and the heartbeat was perfect—a hundred-and-twenty beats per minute.

He apologized and said he would speak to the nurse practitioner about her technique and assured us that he would take over our ultrasounds until we graduate.

We had too many heart-attack moments in the first trimester and I didn't know how much more we could take, but our next ultrasound ended up being the last one before we graduated and again, thankfully, everything was perfect. The baby's heartbeat was up to a hundred-and-sixty beats per minute and its size was measuring a couple of days bigger than where I was at. That was a very happy, happy send-off.

♥ ♡ ♥

A CANDID CONVERSATION WITH RILEY & BOBBI

By: Bobbi and Riley

Bobbi: I wish more people did the work before they became parents, or at least thought about it. For couples like us, you put in the work of thinking about it because it doesn't just happen. We had to sit at a table and get honest with each other and make sure we were on the same page. We were not surprised by the baby; the baby had been planned for in every single way possible. I remember saying, "If we're going to do this, I don't want to adopt, I would like to try to have a baby." I wanted to physically have a baby.

Riley: That was awesome. I was surprised when she said that and it really got me excited. When I told her I wanted a child, it took her some time to process and prepare. I remember her coming home and saying that this is something she was ready to do with me. She said, "I want to do this with you." We sat at the dining room table and she said, "I love you, and this is something that

I want to do with you and I know we'd be great parents together." I remember that because it was a toss-up; it wasn't like a deal-breaker not to have a child, but it was a very pivotal moment in our relationship. We took a step forward in our relationship when we decided to become moms.

I love how we started to do spiritual work together. We did a lot of spiritual work because of the complexities of two women having a child together. We wanted to make sure that we were solid before bringing a child into the world. It was important that our child have a solid foundation.

I strongly believed that you get to define what family is for you. Our family may look different than what we've been told it should be, but we are a family. This is what it looks like for us. We are so very proud!

Bobbi: I am jumping to when we physically started to do the process. I remember being out of town when we started the actual process of this incredible journey. We both were so excited, but then our feet settled and we found a wonderful facility to help us bring this dream to reality. This process was "God" created and we know it!

Riley: Do you remember that morning we prayed together? We like praying in the morning. We prayed to know if this is the right fit for us. Up to this point, honestly, at times it did feel very superficial—it was weird, it felt like picking an outfit...what looks good? We woke up and we prayed and we opened the computer, that's how we knew this was the right union in every way. It was really beautiful and it just felt right. We were incredibly lucky to have such amazing support throughout our journey. The guidance that was around us was nothing short of a blessing!

Bobbi: And honestly, the financial part of it—I don't know if people talk about that—if we focused on that, I can see how it could be stressful and discouraging. I'm just grateful that we trusted the process, we trusted each other, and put one foot in front of the other. We weren't afraid to do everything possible to build our family and we didn't let anything stop us. Our spirituality kept us grounded.

We got pregnant with twins right away and we lost them both by ten weeks. I'm sorry if I'm jumping all around; it's all coming back to me. We lost the twins by ten weeks. I don't know if I was disturbed the way I hear that other people are disturbed, to be quite honest. I don't think about it that often . . . maybe because of the angel we have now. Maybe because I believe everything happens for a reason and we were exactly where we were supposed to be . . . but in the middle of the storm! Was very difficult. I tell our son often, "Thank you for choosing us."

Riley: I remember that you sat on the beach and held your stomach and just . . . you let it out. You don't remember how much it hurt. After the loss, we went on vacation to a very healing place, Tulum, Mexico. When you go there, it's like it just takes all your problems. We needed to get grounded again.

I remember, we came back from Tulum, and I said, "Bobbi, let's just take a break." We agreed to take a long break. Then, you walked in on a Monday, and said, "I'm ready." You just walked into the room. Quiet. It was quiet and you said, "I'm ready. I'm ready to try again."

Bobbi: It felt easier trying again. I didn't realize until we tried later how fortunate we were. For me to get pregnant at forty years old, plus we only went through two rounds of IVF. The first time, I had a miscarriage, and the second time we had our son. I wouldn't change anything in our process, I wouldn't change my spiritual journey, I wouldn't change anything that we did. I thought it was exactly how it's supposed to be to form our family.

Riley: I love that my mom was so on board. I remember seeing her face when our son was born. I could see her looking at me and she gave me this look like, here you go, you're parents now. In our community also, we had so much love and support, because honestly, our whole tribe, all of our people rallied around us. We made our family our way and it is beautiful. The blessings are endless!

I hold on tightly to the memories of my first pregnancy. I cherish all of those amazing feelings because they were some of the most beautiful moments of my life. Every pregnancy after my first one was shrouded in complete fear and anxiety. That first feeling has always stayed with me. I remember that I was happy. That first one, that was amazing.

REFLECTION

"The hardest thing about 'everything happens for a reason' is waiting for that reason to come along."

-Unknown

The art of waiting. Get used to it, because waiting is a huge part of this story. You can't be real about infertility unless you get real about how much of what you will go through is waiting.

We are always waiting. Waiting for appointments, for our period, for our cycle to begin. Waiting to recover from surgeries after discovering polyps, fibroids, or endometriosis. Waiting to start our injections and for the perfect time to do the trigger shot. Waiting by the phone for our test results and blood work. We wait to ask questions of our doctors and we wait for the answers. We wait with a full bladder after a transfer and we wait the excruciating two weeks for the embryo to implant. We wait to see two lines on a stick. We wait, with our breath held, for the first sonogram images, waiting to exhale when we hear a heartbeat. We wait for it to all work, and often we wait to begin again if it all falls apart. We wait to save up more money. We wait to have a normal sex life again. If we are lucky, we wait to "graduate" to OB-GYN. We wait for months and hope that we will get to meet our babies.

We spend most of our time on this journey waiting for the next thing to begin. We can become transfixed on the wait and block out everything else. The wait almost becomes a place of safety as we try to grasp control of the uncontrollable. How much of life do we miss because of waiting? Time is not something that anyone gets back. I don't have any magic answers for how to get through any of this; I can't tell you how to make it all work out. I just know that you have to try to remember the life you had before getting thrown onto the infertility train. I bet it was full and vibrant and complete, even if you didn't have the child that you so desperately wanted. You deserve an incredible life. You deserved it before infertility hit and you deserve it after everything you've gone through. We make so many plans, schedules, and charts dealing with IUI or IVF, we have to remember that a major part of the plan has to be continuing to live our lives. Our very best lives. You are complete now just the way you are, and you are enough, with or without a child.

Chapter Five

MISCARRIAGE:
Why is My Body Betraying Me?

"I will always wonder who you would have been . . ."

-Unknown

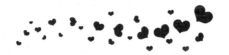

There is nothing I avoid more than talking about my miscarriage. Maybe that is the problem. Nobody wants to talk about it, so no one is even remotely prepared when it happens. In 2018, during an interview with Robin Roberts for *Good Morning America*, Michelle Obama opened up about her miscarriage. "I felt like I failed because I didn't know how common miscarriages were because we don't talk about them," Obama said. "We sit in our own pain, thinking that somehow we're broken . . . that's one of the reasons why I think it's important to talk to young mothers about the fact that miscarriages happen."[1]

Nothing in my life was as painful as the loss of a wanted child. My miscarriage didn't just hurt, it consumed me with pain, disbelief, anguish, and utter devastation. It was like I became a dysfunctional version of Humpty Dumpty—I fell off the wall and nothing could put me back together again. It was a foul and complete disruption of my life. I didn't know that anything could hurt like that, and I didn't know how to find a way out of the sadness. My miscarriage felt like the biggest betrayal my body could make. My heart hurts now spilling it all out here on the page. For a long time, I felt like I was slowly suffocating under

---

1   Katie Kinderlan et al. "Michelle Obama opens up about her miscarriage, going through IVF and Donald Trump in ABC News primetime special for new memoir 'Becoming,'" Good Morning America, November 9, 2018. https://www.goodmorningamerica.com/culture/story/michelle-obama-opens-miscarriage-ivf-donald-trump-abc-59033287

the weight of my unhappiness. Time alone does not erase the feelings of sadness. You don't simply snap out of grief and sorrow and then return to being whole. Beginning to heal takes a lot of support and a lot of effort.

Looking back, all I remember before the miscarriage was the total and complete elation of being pregnant. I was glowing from the inside out, radiating from every pore with the glory of pregnancy and the life inside of me. I reveled in every single moment of morning sickness because it was proof of what was happening inside of me. I loved being pregnant. I loved it more than I can adequately express in these pages. I felt so powerful and so beautiful. I was strong and perfectly complete in those weeks. I didn't think anything could go wrong. I had survived two unsuccessful IVF attempts and now I had success. I thought, in my ignorant bliss, that nothing could go wrong because I had done all the hard work and done all the right things. I did my yoga, took my prenatals, stopped drinking coffee, endured acupuncture (and that nasty tea that went with it). I took the shots and followed all the rules. I had paid the full price of admission to motherhood so now it was my time to enjoy life.

There is an amazing vividness to the day when it all came crashing down—I remember every step I took and everything I did that day from the moment I woke up. It was December, so the holidays were in full effect. I went to the Apple Store to pick up an iPad I'd had engraved for my husband. It said, "Merry Christmas, I love you Papa, Love Baby Trinchieri." I remember being so excited for my husband to open it up on Christmas Day. His first gift as a father; his first gift from his child. I remember picking up a vegetarian sandwich with extra avocado for myself for dinner and doing gentle pregnancy yoga poses that night to stretch and relax. I remember sitting in bed and settling in to read a book about babies and motherhood. Then, I remember feeling something warm and wet in my pajamas. I got up to go to the bathroom, not nervous because I felt no pain. The successful IVF cycle had given me a false sense that I was invincible. I was pregnant, life was good. I didn't have a sense that anything was wrong. I don't remember what I thought I was going to see, but I know I never expected to see blood. At first just a little, but then a rush and constant flow. I can still hear the inhuman cry I made involuntarily. Then the cry turned into a scream. My husband ran into the bathroom and stared hopelessly, frozen in the door. "I'm bleeding, I'm bleeding," I kept crying out, over and over. So much blood. I couldn't get up from the toilet. Tommaso left to go to the twenty-four-hour drug store to get maxi pads. While he was gone, I stayed on the toilet holding myself and crying bitter tears of loss and pain, feeling complete anguish and completely helpless.

When Tommaso got back, I called my doctor and Tommaso started googling. He was looking for some sort of verification that what we both knew was happening wasn't really happening. My doctor tried to calm me down. I will forever be grateful that I had an amazing doctor who called me back after midnight when he heard my frantic message that I was bleeding. He told me that it could be a blood clot, he had noticed one on my last ultrasound. He told me that sometimes bleeding was common. He wanted me to try and relax and to come into his office at 7:00 a.m., before it opened, so he could examine me. He tried to reassure me that everything could be okay. I tried and tried to hold on to even the tiniest sliver of hope. I wanted to believe so much that it would work out. I didn't sleep a wink that night, neither did Tommaso. He held me in his arms as I cried. I was still awake at 4:00 a.m. when my doctor called me back to see if I was still bleeding. I was. I had never seen so much blood in my life. I filled pad after pad. It never seemed to stop. I was still bleeding at my appointment the next morning. I sat in that waiting room, knowing that I had lost my pregnancy. Even with that knowledge, I wasn't prepared for the intense pain that hit me when the doctor told me in a heavy and broken voice that he no longer saw signs of a pregnancy. It was all gone, all my hope and happiness, and all my dreams of the child that I could have had. If the human capacity for love is endless, so is the capacity for pain. I had never hurt so much in my life. My sadness was an endless void. Aside from my wedding day, my first miscarriage was the only time I had ever seen my husband break down and cry. I was lying in bed and crying into my pillow while my husband took on the tough job of calling our parents and delivering the news. I heard his voice break and a huge sob escaped. He hung up and collapsed on the bed next to me and cried. There are no accurate words for what we lost that day, and that was only the first miscarriage.

♥ ♡ ♥

THERE'S NO FIRST PLACE IN THE PAIN OLYMPICS

By: Maya

My daughter was born via embryo donation in March 2015, then about two years later, I got pregnant naturally. I was shocked! I had done IUI, IVF, and egg donation before we landed on embryo donation as the way to build our family, so getting pregnant naturally somehow felt like I beat the system. It was like, "Take that, infertility!" It felt so validating. I had never been pregnant naturally and we weren't trying either. I honestly don't know how it happened.

It was New Year's Eve when I took the pregnancy test—I took five of them because I was thinking this can't be real. When we saw the heartbeat around seven or eight weeks, we said "Wow, maybe this is really happening." We had always wanted two children, and we genuinely felt like this was it!

It was Valentine's Day when we went back for the next check-up. We were sitting in the waiting room for a while, hearing all these heartbeats through the different exam room doors. I looked at my husband and thought, *I have a really bad feeling.* I didn't want to say it, but I didn't feel like I felt at ten or eleven weeks the first time around. I kept thinking, *Maybe it's a boy and it feels different.* I was trying to tell myself everything I possibly could to settle my nerves. *We're okay, we're okay, we're okay.* I went into the exam room and did the abdominal ultrasound and I had this image of a floating, lifeless mass in my uterus. Before, even at just seven weeks or whatever it was, we saw subtle movements of life. An energy and vibration. This baby . . . wasn't moving. There was no heartbeat and it was this heavy, lifeless thing, floating inside of me. I remember the silence that was broken by the sound of my gasp, then tears. Raw anguish, shock, and sadness burst out of my face. My doctor was as great as one can be in those hard moments. With my daughter, I'd had a really hard delivery and he saved my life. I loved and trusted this man. He was flustered for a minute and I could see he didn't want this outcome to be true. He quickly moved to the vaginal ultrasound and said, "Wait, wait, let me just see, let me try one more thing." He did the other ultrasound and there was nothing. I remember he left the room saying, "This is the part of my job that I hate, I'll give you a second." He left the room and I cried.

Then, it became all about the game plan. What are we going to do? Am I going to go home and bleed out in a bathtub with my two-year-old there? I was still nursing her—was that why this baby didn't survive? Then came the moment when I started to blame myself; how could I find reasons why this is my fault?

I don't know why our brain goes there, but it often does, and you have to tell yourself: I did nothing wrong. You have to keep telling yourself that this happens and we're all doing the best that we can, and it's awful. As a psychotherapist working primarily with fertility patients, I go through miscarriages and losses of wanted pregnancies with my clients all the time it never gets easier. It's not the pain Olympics—no one wins. There are so many different kinds of losses with infertility: The loss of being able to make a baby in the privacy of your own home rather than a doctor's office; the loss you feel when embryos don't make it to a viable stage of development; the loss of genetic heritage or being able to carry your child; miscarriage and stillbirth—there are all these shades of grief and loss.

I ended up having a D&C (Dilation and Curettage) the next day. I thought, *I'm not playing this game.* I'd heard too many stories of people experiencing really traumatizing miscarriages and I was not emotionally prepared for that trauma. The D&C was quick and totally surreal. I recovered. We said goodbye in the way that we could.

Now, we are legitimately not trying to get pregnant and we're very happy with our family of three, but it isn't what I imagined. There's this constant revision of the story. I often talk about the gap between expectations and reality with my clients. There is often a *huge* gap between what we wanted or expected and what actually happens and it takes time for the head and the heart to come to terms with all of it. Right now, I'm so grateful for the family we have and that we were able to survive the very dark "journey to parenthood."

Tommaso and I told ourselves that next time it would be different. We would be ready and so much more prepared. "So, you had a miscarriage," they all said, "They are so common for first pregnancies, next time . . . next time it will all be fine." So we prepared differently. Acupuncture was now twice a week; fertility yoga was every night. I began a special diet and started seeing a therapist so I would be calm and serene at all times. We told no one, that way—as we so smugly thought, there would be no one to un-tell if for some reason the transfer didn't work out. That first time, everyone knew, and I had miscarried so quickly that people were still offering me congratulations at work, forcing me to have to explain again and again what happened. We lied to ourselves that telling other people is what made it all so hard. This time, we were doing it right.

It started so perfectly. I did my two-week wait on total bed rest. Our numbers from all the blood draws were solid. We were measuring growth and our embryo seemed to be settling in sweetly. I stayed on modified bed rest after the initial two weeks: I went from bed, to bathroom, to kitchen, to the doctor's office. Last time was a fluke. This was our baby. This time we would be fine.

Then one night, I had a horrible dream. It was so un-settling that it jolted me awake at 4:30 in the morning and it hung over me so heavily that I was not able to get back to sleep. I had dreamed, in vivid detail, that I had another miscarriage. When Tommaso woke up a few hours later, I shared my terrible nightmare. "It's OK," he reassured me. "Everything is OK, you are still thinking about the last time. This is different, everything is good. You'll be fine." I think he knew too that something felt off.

I had no pain. I had no cramps. I just had this horri-ble, nagging feeling deep down that something was very wrong. I wasn't surprised or alarmed when I felt some-thing wet on my pajamas later that night. I didn't even have to check to know that it was blood. I knew. I knew what my body and my baby had tried to tell me during the night. I was not pregnant anymore.

All the thoughts we had of how much easier it would be this time around flew out the door. It hurt just as much to lose another pregnancy as it had the first time. While we didn't have anyone to un-tell, we had plenty of people that needed to be informed about my miscarriage after the fact. There is no "better" or "easier" way to navigate through a completely messed up situation.

I was further along in this pregnancy and, after a few days, we discovered that my body hadn't been able to complete the miscarriage naturally. I had to schedule a D&C. It is excruciating to sit in your doctor's waiting room among smiling moms and healthy, growing bellies while you are waiting in silence for the doctor to remove the final traces of everything you had spent so long hop-ing for and wanting so much.

There were miscarriages after this as well and they all blur into each other. I was numb and going through the motions. I blocked out the pain, not because I didn't feel, because I felt too much. I still had so much hope and it got crushed with each loss. My hope became tempered with the knowledge that it was all so very fragile. I was in a whirlwind of trying to equally measure my desire to keep trying and the threshold of my pain. I am still not sure if those things are ever measurable. What I do know for sure is that if you are infertile, you are never presented with easy choices.

♥ ♡ ♥

HIS BIRTHDAY WAS YESTERDAY . . .

By: Stephanie

Every year, on August 26th, I relive one of the worst moments in my life. I was such a positive person before I lost my son. I'm still a positive person, but I'm cautiously optimistic now. I woke up on August 25th, 2010, took a shower, and started getting ready for work. I was running late, as usual, and then I felt a gush: my water had broken. I was nowhere near my due date; I was twenty-four weeks. I was terrified, but I remained positive that everything would be okay. I rushed myself to the hospital, then my doctor transferred me back downtown via ambulance to the hospital that specializes in early deliveries. Still, I thought if I listened to the doctors and kept calm, everything would be okay. Liam would just spend some time in a NICU. We could visit him, I would pump milk for him . . .

I stayed in the hospital overnight and a young, sweet nurse would come in to check on his heartbeat—she would do a little dance to his heartbeat. I always felt reassured after her visits. It was a long night of terror mixed with hope listening to my little boy's heartbeat. At some point early in the morning, they decided to get him out, they didn't want to risk sepsis. I was on board. I remember lying there, strapped to the table, with the anesthesiologist asking me if I was feeling any pain. I remember the nurse coming around the table to show me a golf-ball-sized fibroid. The next time, it was the doctor who came around. He told me Liam was gone . . . Tom tells me I howled and tried to get up from the table. The anesthesiologist immediately put me under and everything went white. I saw a white teddy bear, a white mobile of circus animals, a completely white nursery with lots of cribs, and I somehow knew Liam was there, but also, I knew that was where he was going to stay. The next thing I remember was the doctors coming into my hospital room. I was finally able to hold my beautiful, big-eyed (during my ultrasounds all the techs made comments on how big Liam's eyes were) baby boy in my arms, and the doctor who had tried to intubate him was crying next to my bed. Upon leaving, they handed me a bear that was the same weight as an average newborn to take home. I hated that bear. It was a heavy reminder of my loss but I wouldn't dream of giving it away.

I don't remember much in between that day and Liam's memorial. Most of my family came to say goodbye to him. I am so lucky to have such a supportive and loving family. My cousin Candace gave me a painting of strawberries that still hangs in our kitchen. During pregnancy, strawberries were all Liam and I wanted to eat. The one thing I remember clearly is standing in our kitchen under that very painting, sobbing in Tom's arms saying, "I just want to be a mom." We went to grief counseling and met some wonderful people who all shared some variation of the loss of a child, from the first few weeks of pregnancy to hours after birth. It was tremendously helpful to grieve with a group of people going through the same experience. I am so proud of my cousin for sharing her own heartbreaking experience, allowing us all to honor our lost children in her book, and being a wonderful advocate for us.

Weeks later, we went to see my OB-GYN. She walked into the room and absent-mindedly asked us how the baby was doing. She was a great doctor and had many, many, many patients—she was also human and immediately realized her error. It still stung, of course, but I wouldn't trade her for another OB—she was fantastic! I was forty-two when I gave birth to Liam, so we talked about what was next. We discussed my pregnancy with Liam and how much it had hurt all the time; I always felt like I was in the throes of PMS and on the verge of starting my period. No morning sickness, just cramps and discomfort. Diagnosis: most likely an irritable uterus. We came up with a plan to incorporate progesterone injections when it was safe for me to get pregnant again. She asked us to wait at least ten months, and that twelve would be better. So, in the meantime I started planning our wedding; my type-A personality was in full throttle mode and it kept me from sobbing all the time.

July 16th, 2011: our big day had arrived! I was exhausted after all the wedding planning and preparation! But it was a wonderful distraction that had allowed me to slowly heal and come to terms with the loss. I had infused Liam into our wedding ceremony. While I'm not a particularly religious person, I know I will see him again, and I knew then that his spirit was with us, at least in my heart. I remember standing at the altar facing Tom while holding his hands and our minister was talking about how our hands would someday hold our children. Out of nowhere, it seemed this sense of utter euphoria took over me, the air around me swirled, and I felt a presence move through my body. A friend of mine said butterflies were flying around us as if released on cue. It was him—in my heart of hearts, I knew it was Liam! Little did we know ...

The next morning, I woke up in our honeymoon suite before Tom, as usual, since he's the night owl in our relationship. I went to the bathroom and started digging around in my diddy bag for my toothbrush and came across a pregnancy test I had stashed in there a few months prior. On a whim, I decided to use it since we started trying again at eleven months—not ten, not twelve, but at eleven months. I could not believe my eyes, I was pregnant!! I rushed to tell Tom and we both concluded it was the best wedding present ever. I never look at butterflies as just butterflies anymore. To me, they are Liam coming to see me or sending me messages. I look at my wedding photos and in most of them I have my hand over my belly—it blows me away.

My pregnancy with Gracie was one-hundred-dred-percent different. I had serious morning sickness and absolutely no cramps. The normalcy of this pregnancy helped me heal even further from Liam's death; it allowed me to remove the blame I put on myself and to accept that maybe Liam was supposed to stay in that big white nursery? Maybe those big eyes saw and knew something I didn't? Maybe I love Gracie even more because of him? I don't know, but maybe when I see him again, I will. Needless to say, I was scared out of my mind for the entire pregnancy with Grace. I did not enjoy being pregnant at all, although, when she started to kick my heart was triggered into having a little more hope. We started progesterone in the second or third trimester, I don't recall exactly. I was on bed rest the last three weeks and my wonderful doctor allowed me to get many, many ultrasounds of Gracie, even a 3D ultrasound. On March 8th, 2012, I had a scheduled C-section to deliver Gracie. During the C-section, I was still terrified; it wasn't until I heard her cry, felt her little body resting on my chest, and looked into her eyes that I completely let go of my fears. She was here, *really* here! My little rainbow baby. Finally, at forty-four, I was a mommy. Oh, and that bear I took home from the hospital? Gracie loves "heavy bear" and he sleeps with her every night.

I will never forget you Liam and it is a given that I will always love you. Until we meet again, I'll keep an eye out for butterflies.

HOW I BECAME AN IVF AND FERTILITY COACH

By: Monica

I was born in Colombia, South America. At the age of thirty-two, my husband and I were informed that my fallopian tubes were blocked due to severe endometriosis. Even after doing a laparoscopy to try and unblock them, I couldn't get pregnant. IVF was the only option. My husband Moshe was supportive all the way, however, the emotional stress was very heavy on both of us. My first cycle was successful: they retrieved thirty-four eggs and fourteen fertilized. Four of the eggs were transferred and suddenly I became a mom. My girl is now thirteen years old.

We decided to have a second baby. I thought it was so easy the first time around, so I assumed another cycle would be the same. It was not.

Due to a mistake made by the clinic in the dosage of medicine, I got OHSS. My ovaries were so swollen and painful they were leaking fluid into my body. The cycle had to be canceled. We were lucky, the reproductive endocrinologist offered us another cycle at no cost, assuming their full responsibility for this mistake.

The next time, we decided to do chromosomal testing, because we wanted a baby boy. Out of four embryos, three were male and the single female embryo was not quite as developed. We decided to transfer all four. Oddly enough, we got pregnant with that baby girl.

My whole pregnancy was good—very uneventful, even the amniocentesis, which confirmed that we were expecting a girl. Everything was normal; no one knew I was developing a blood issue. At thirty-nine weeks, three days before the delivery due date, my baby girl, Isabelle, died in my womb due to a blood clot in the umbilical cord. I had to deliver her anyway. Devastated and lost, and overwhelmed with a deep sense of guilt for what happened, we wasted no time pursuing a fourth round of IVF less than two months later. I got a positive test, but from the sadness, the loss, the stress, and the fear, combined with other personal issues, I miscarried at seven weeks.

By this time, Moshe and I were completely lost, showing no sign of how to find our way back to one another again. Driven by fear, immense pain, and ego, our relationship turned into a disaster and we almost got divorced. We had to choose to make some changes. We chose love.

In 2012, we decided to go for another round of IVF, our fifth and final. This cycle was an amazing experience. It was full of love, healthy dialogue, and peace—a direct result of the internal struggles and the shifts we made, together, as a team. This last round of IVF resulted in another girl who is now six years old. Everything I went through led me to be an IVF, fertility, and life coach, and the author of a book to help others organize their journey through IVF with love and positivity.

Do you notice from reading these stories that there is no one way to deal with grief? There is no guidebook to tell you what is appropriate and there is no such thing as right or wrong. It can be hard not to project onto others how you think you would react, in any situation. I try never to minimize another's pain and, more importantly, I try not to be dismissive of my own pain. Loss is loss, and it may hit you in ways that surprise you. Never feel guilty about the pain you experience. Grieving doesn't make you weak, it makes you human. And, hope is eternal.

STILL WAITING FOR
OUR HAPPY ENDING

By: Saima (United Kingdom)

It's been a long journey and I'm still walking it. It's been eight years now. When we got married, children were one of those things we knew we wanted. Six months into trying, I felt that something was not quite right. I remember my husband saying to me, "You're fine, you just need to relax, it's okay." I was thinking, *No, it's not okay.* I was making a mental list, *Let's go to the doctor, let's sort a diet out.* You know how easy it is to become obsessed with it all. You start Googling everything. It's like you know there's a problem and you have to convince other people that something is off. I thought, *Let's go to the consultation, see what's going on, and what the options are for us.*

We both got tested and all of the test results revealed an unexplained infertility diagnosis. We immediately started the IVF process and after my egg retrieval, I fell pregnant naturally. I was thinking, *Wow, Grace of God, this is good, everything is great.* Nine weeks into the pregnancy, I had a silent miscarriage; my body was still telling me I was pregnant even though the pregnancy had ended. At nine weeks, I went for my scan: there was no heartbeat and I had to have it surgically removed. Even then I knew that many women miscarry in their first pregnancy—it was sad and it hurt, but it wasn't unheard of. I had fallen pregnant naturally so it was all going to be fine. We both came to terms with it. We still had eggs and embryos from the IVF process; we still had hope.

In 2016, I fell pregnant again naturally with our son. I developed gestational diabetes, but otherwise, everything is quite controlled. When you've miscarried in the past, you become a little more paranoid about things. I was extra careful with what I ate, cutting out absolutely everything I thought was problematic. When I became diabetic, I was even more careful. I had to go in every week to get tested to make sure my levels were right. Every other week I went for scans. I was very careful. They told me they were going to book me at thirty-six weeks to be induced because I was very high risk with a previous miscarriage and diabetes.

I was fine for the whole pregnancy. On Monday, the fifth of December, my water broke, a week before I was to be induced. It was six in the morning and I said to my husband, "Our waters are broken." At this stage, we were excited and I was feeling fine. The baby had been moving, we had no concerns. We went to the hospital and I called my sister and said, "This is it!" We were all excited.

As we got to the hospital, I found I was bleeding. It was my first pregnancy, so I was thinking, *Is this normal? Is it the mucus plug?* I certainly didn't feel like there was anything wrong. When we checked in, based on the reaction of the nurses, I gathered that there was a problem. I am a matter-of-fact person, so if there's a situation, my emotions get set aside and I deal with the situation that is at hand. So, when we were told, "There is no heartbeat and unfortunately he's passed away," my automatic reaction was, *What do we do now?* My husband is quite the opposite. He was devastated, as you can imagine. He was asking, "Are we hearing the right news? Can we get a second opinion?" We got the second opinion of course but, as a woman, you kind of know. You know your own body; you know something has happened.

So, then they tell me that I am in labor and that I will need to deliver. I remember telling them, "No, that's not going to happen. You might as well arrange a C-section because this is not happening." They explained to me that I was already very dilated and just needed to deliver. I remember looking at my husband and saying, "They are telling me to deliver," and he nodded his head yes. So, I was in full labor, my husband was making phone calls and telling family. Everyone was devastated for us. The labor was long. From seven in the morning until almost midnight. I don't remember pushing but it was me, the force, and the One above, I guess, helping me through it all.

Finally, I delivered. The cord was wrapped around his neck. I guess when the waters broke he got compressed and wrapped in the cord. So, they took the little man away, and next my health was in jeopardy. My body was in shock; I needed transfusions and surgery for a third-degree tear. It was a lot. We had the little man overnight with us. I come from a background where we do burial very quickly, so that morning we had a small window for family to come see him and then they left and we had time alone with him. We had to register his birth and register his death as well. My health started going downhill again. I was having a bad reaction to the blood transfusions and had to be rushed into the Intensive Care Unit. So, my poor husband was burying our child and not knowing if his wife would make it. After three days, I was able to leave the hospital only to come back a few days later with a blood clot in my chest. It was a very traumatic week for us.

After all of this, I started coming to terms with the fact that things are written—if it's meant to be, it's meant to be. I have always felt that way about this journey.

Six months later, I fell pregnant again naturally and at ten weeks, I had another silent miscarriage. So, I was back in surgery again. Two weeks after that, I needed yet another surgery because they had not removed everything and my body still thought I was pregnant. I remember coming out of one of my post-surgery appointments thinking, *That's it, we have these frozen embryos, let's not wait.* I'm sure my husband thought I was crazy, but the embryos were there and I was ready.

So, we started the IVF process again. I was preparing my body, the injections, the meds—you really do structure your whole life around the process. We did a successful transfer and I got pregnant again, but nine weeks later I had another miscarriage. We took a small break and after some time, we are ready to try again. This time the transfer did not take. That felt devastating. I had always fallen pregnant, even naturally, so when it didn't take, that was very hard. We were asking ourselves, *What's going on? What category did I fit in?* I tick all the boxes: I can get pregnant, I can give birth, where exactly do I fit? We were all out of frozen embryos at this point.

I am currently on my third IVF cycle. We don't know yet if we will do a fresh or frozen cycle. Right now, we are getting ready for my egg retrieval. So, we will see . . . we are still praying for our rainbow baby.

REFLECTION

"Grief is like the ocean, it comes in waves, ebbing and flowing. Sometimes the water is calm, and sometimes it is overwhelming. All we can do is learn to swim."

-Vicki Harrison

The difficulty for me in writing a personal reflection on miscarriage is that it still hurts so damn much. Almost a decade later, the wounds are still as fresh and as raw as if it happened only yesterday. The hurt is too much and the cut is too deep to look back and reflect objectively on my experience. I am still coming to terms with my losses and still working on finding some peace within myself. Grief comes and goes in my life like waves in an ocean. Sometimes I can tell my story and not shed a tear; I can talk or write for hours about my whole experience. There are also times when I can't make the words leave my lips and I cry before I even start speaking. It never hits the same way twice. Every day, I experience my loss differently. Every day, I process my loss differently.

There hasn't been some kind of magic moment or event that made my pain stop. I am, years later, still trying to make sense of the senseless, and that's okay. For me, it starts with being loving and forgiving to myself. Taking a deep breath every day and acknowledging that I am still working through all my stuff. I don't have to force myself to forget, I don't have to snap out of it, and, most importantly, I don't have to pretend that I am always fine. I can allow myself to feel all the feelings. So often, I have been forced to be the strong Black woman. It was so much easier and less messy to say I was fine than to try to explain my pain. I now know that vulnerability is not weakness. Being honest about what you feel is what gives you strength. So I say in power, I've had multiple miscarriages. Each loss hurt deeply and I have never been the same again. I am a mother to a son I love more than life itself, and I will never forget any of my children that came before him. They were wished for, wanted, and very loved. They passed on after a brief moment with me, but they were mine and they will always be missed.

Chapter Six

BIRTH:
The Day We've Been Waiting for . . .

*"Giving birth should be your
greatest achievement, not your
greatest fear."*

-Jane Weidman

Birth is big business. Millions of advertising dollars are spent annually telling us about the wonders and joys of having a baby. Women can be thrown off by the differences between the idealization of giving birth and the raw reality of what actually happens. I am not only talking about having different experiences based on your race and the bias you might face in the medical industry—giving birth is different from what women have been told to expect. There is even a trend to reject media that might show that reality to women. In 2020, the ABC television network rejected a commercial for airing during the Oscars because it accurately depicted postpartum reality and was therefore deemed too graphic. The Frida Mom commercial "begins with a baby's cry and a tired new mom turning on her lamp and rising from bed. She's wearing a tank top, mesh underwear and a large pad and is clearly still recovering from giving birth. She waddles to the bathroom with the pain of postpartum recovery and refills a peri bottle, a plastic squirt bottle that new moms use for toileting hygiene after giving birth. She's wincing, she's bleeding, she's in pain and she's very, very real."[1]

---

1   Heather Marcoux, "This refreshingly honest postpartum commercial was rejected from TV," *Motherly,* February 7, 2020. https://www.mother.ly/news/this-is-the-frida-mom-ad-the-oscars-banned

In 2019, the same telecast had accepted and aired an ad featuring a close-up of a beautifully made-up woman in front of a white screen talking about the fact that her military husband overseas was able to virtually attend the birth of their child with the magic of a cell phone video. The message is loud and clear. You can talk about the miracle of birth, but under no circumstances do you show a broad audience the actual experience. If you don't know, how do you prepare? If you are white with money, support, and society on your side, and even you don't know the reality, then where does that leave women of color in the racial hierarchy of motherhood? If white women are lied to about the birth experience, the fact that women of color are further marginalized can make us feel that we are not important at all. "In fact, the reality presented in the Frida Mom commercial is exactly what America needs to see right now. For too long we've been ignoring what recovery from birth is really like. And when we ignore how hard postpartum recovery is it is easier to normalize sending working moms back to their job within a few weeks of giving birth or forcing recovering mothers to resume unpaid labor by denying them support during this critical time."[2] In the United States, your birth experience depends not just on your race but also on your socioeconomic level. The reverence and privilege of the grand and beautiful birth experience and postpartum recovery are seen through a very economic lens. The more money and status you have, the more you are granted postpartum reprieve. Honestly, the existing maternity leave policy is so stingy that it's practically non-existent. Our system forces many women back into the workforce immediately after giving birth, and this is so commonplace in America that we don't even question its absurdity.

---

2   Marcoux, "This refreshingly honest postpartum commercial..."

I adopted my son from birth. Choosing open adoption meant that we had a relationship with his birth mom. She found the adoption profile my husband and I had set up online through our adoption agency and emailed me. I was driving when I saw the notification pop-up on my phone, showing that I had a message from our adoption profile. I have never pulled over so quickly in my entire life. I emailed back and within a few hours we had our first phone call with the incredible woman who would be Max's birth mom. Having her choose us to be Max's parents was the equivalent of every holiday celebration rolled into one. She was early enough in her pregnancy that I was able to be present during his ultrasound at fourteen weeks. I heard Max's heartbeat and found out he was a boy.

That ultrasound appointment was our first meeting. Remember how I often talk about expectation versus reality? Well, I don't know exactly how I thought our first meeting would happen, but I didn't think it would be me alone in the parking lot of the doctor's office crying and shoving a huge bouquet of flowers into the birth mom's hands. That's right, I met the biological mother of my son in a parking lot before going in for her ultrasound appointment. She was twenty years younger than me, white, and she had a lovely bump. I'm sure we made an odd couple sitting together nervously in the waiting room. I had flown to the East Coast alone since Tommaso couldn't get the time off of work. However calm and measured I prepared myself to be, I was an emotional mess. I had never heard a heartbeat in any of my pregnancies. I always miscarried in the first trimester and then found out that there was no heartbeat at the ultrasound appointment. I wanted to be so respectful of her and her pregnancy. Even though we were going to be adopting Max, it was one-hundred-percent her pregnancy and I never wanted to lose sight of that fact. In that moment, when the lights were dimmed in the room and all of a sudden I heard that quick and beautiful sound of the beating heart, I melted into a big mess. She was pregnant, but for the first time, I witnessed that moment. I had *my* moment. I got to hear my child's heartbeat and it was the most beautiful sound in the world. I couldn't help myself. I broke down crying. Hearing a heartbeat, the thing that I had always been denied in my quest for motherhood, was like finally coming up for air and taking a deep inhalation after being submerged in water for a long time. I was so emotional that her boyfriend tried to comfort me. The technician asked if we wanted to know the sex. She looked at me and I nodded. "It's a boy," the tech told us. Without hesitation, his birth mom looked me squarely in the eye and said, "So, what are you naming your son?" It was that moment, that I fully and completely became Max's mom. She gave me ownership not just in that moment, but in all the moments I never thought I would have as someone who was infertile. She gave me all the moments to be his mom.

Tommaso and I were in the room with her when she gave birth at 1:35 p.m. on a February afternoon. She had called us the night before at 8:45 p.m. and told us that she was having contractions. Since this was her third pregnancy, she was completely calm and let us know it was going to be a long time before she went to the hospital. I think I dropped the phone and suppressed a scream of joy. I was so excited to tell Tommaso, but since we had a house full of expectant grandparents, we wanted to keep the news to ourselves until we left for the hospital. For the rest of the night, the two of us silently laughed together and shared secret smiles. We went up to bed and stared at one another, our smiles almost breaking our faces. Was this really happening? Was this the moment our lives would shift forever and we would be having a baby?

The next call came at 4:08 a.m. I don't remember drifting off to sleep, but I must have because the call woke me up and I bolted out of bed like a shot. "Meet us at the hospital," she told me. We were there in record time. We arrived at the hospital so quickly that we were waiting in the lobby for her when she drove up. I was nervous, Tommaso seemed to be walking around the hospital room in a daze, and I recall how calm she was and how comforting that felt. I know it took hours but everything seemed to happen in a rush, like I inhaled deeply and let it all out suddenly in a powerful whoosh. She got her epidural, she began to push. I held one of her legs. Suddenly, there was Max, screaming at the indignity of suddenly leaving his dark, warm home of nine months and being thrust out into the world. I actually cut the umbilical cord. I watched with love as she did skin to skin contact with Max when he finally emerged and they placed him on her chest. Then I held him. After more than four years, I held my child in my arms.

One of my most cherished possessions is the photo of my son and his birth mother luxuriating in the beautiful moments after his birth in their private skin-to-skin contact. She held him to her chest whispering to him. I never asked what she said and I will never know, but I do know in my heart that Max heard her and loved her. That moment was one of the most beautiful things I have ever witnessed in my life. I cherish that photo because I know that one day I will show it to Max. He will be able to witness the proof that, without a doubt, he came into the world surrounded by so much love. The relationship we have with his birth mother may not be the relationship we all dreamed about, but the love we all feel for Max has never waivered. I can't express fully the gratitude and adoration I feel for the beautiful young woman who carried and loved Max enough to trust me and choose me to be his mother. She came into our lives like a shooting star— bright, hot, and illuminating our hearts. She fulfilled our greatest dream of becoming parents. Again, I say it because I can never say it enough: she was able to do what nothing in modern medicine was ever able to achieve. She made me a mother. For that, I am forever grateful. I also remind myself daily of the amount of love it took for her to place the beautiful boy she just delivered into my arms. My best day on this earth may have been one of her most painful. I carry that with me.

Later that day, when Tommaso and I left the hospital to get a quick dinner, we sat at the table in the loud, gaudy chain restaurant close to the hospital, staring at one another over a platter of fried shrimp and fries. I don't know which one of us ordered it, because neither of us was eating anything. We sat in silence, completely shaken to our core. Our entire world had changed. Our lives would never be the same. It was a new beginning. At the same time, how could we ever shake off and forget everything that happened to get us to this place? How do we begin a new chapter when it felt like we had been completely broken along the way? So, we sat and stared at one another, both embracing so many feelings, so many deep emotions, so much disbelief. Silently counting the times we had our hopes dashed in this journey. Almost afraid to truly believe, afraid to begin to contemplate our complete happiness. Then my husband looked me in the eye and simply said, "We're parents." Then the tears came, then the smiles, then the loud laughter that grew even louder and more obnoxious because no one in the restaurant would ever understand our inside joke. We gathered up our coats, paid our bill, and went back to the hospital to hold our son.

Even in the beauty of that magical day when Max was born, racism raised its nasty head. My husband and I are an interracial couple. Max's biological parents happened to be an interracial couple as well, only in that instance his birth mother was white and the biological father was Black. She was young and on public assistance, giving birth in a southern hospital not used to dealing with open adoption scenarios. The undercurrent of racism that the doctors and nurses had toward a white woman placing her child for adoption with a Black mom was palpable. It went beyond the glances and loud, incredulous whispers. It got to the point that when Tommaso and I visited the hospital room after Max was delivered, the nurses would remove Max from the room and not bring him back while we were there. Even with the legal papers that stated we were the adoptive parents, the hospital refused to issue us parental bracelets allowing us access to the nursery. Our lawyer had to call the Hospital Director before we were acknowledged as parents. In a blatant move that was illegal, several nurses spoke to Max's birth mom and attempted to get her to change her mind about the adoption. Fortunately, we had several months to build a connection and genuine relationship with Max's birth mom. I had even moved across the country for the last month of her pregnancy to better support her and help her get to her doctor's appointments before she delivered. She was able to navigate the nasty tone at the hospital with amazing grace. At one point, she sat up in her bed and exclaimed, "These are his parents, if you have questions, speak to them." If we hadn't built a relationship, if she had not been strong in her convictions, how might that time in a racially charged setting have changed all of our lives?

That time in the hospital with Max's birth mom was also a glaring display of how much economic class plays into the birth experience. Your experience is determined by how much money you have to spend and when you are on public assistance, comfort does not seem high on the list of priorities. When you are Black, no matter what your economic level, the disparities in care still affect your experience. Actress Jodie Turner-Smith labored for four days at home before she gave birth because, as she said, "We had already decided on a home birth because of concerns about negative birth outcomes for Black women in America."[3]

Long before Max was born, I read an article in the Huffington Post from the blog, *YourBrownBaby.com*. It was titled "Birthing While Black: An Experience I Will Never Forget," by Denene Millner. That article impacted me deeply and, after my own experience when Max was born, the article imprinted on me even more. Millner detailed her painful and racially-charged birth experience in a New York Hospital, one that she had chosen for her delivery specifically because they offered a unique VIP Birth Experience. But the hospital betrayed its commitment to fairness by constantly antagonizing Millner with racism—from the unauthorized drug test they gave her child after birth, to being openly incredulous that her partner was by her side, to not even believing that she had actually paid the money for the private birthing suite, the catered dinner, and all the other amenities in the VIP experience.

Denene Millner shared her pain in a *Huffington Post* article, "I wondered then what I know to be true now: It didn't matter how much money I had in my bank account or how good my insurance was, or that I had a ring on my finger, or that I was smart and accomplished, or that I tried to pay my way out of substandard service. At the end of the day, to almost everyone in that hospital, I was just another Black girl pushing out another Black baby and neither of us deserved to be treated with dignity or respect, much less special. That human beings charged with caring for new life and the people who ushered in that miracle could traffic in this kind of reprehensible treatment of anyone, much less a new mother—no matter her race, financial or marital status, or background—is beyond my level of comprehension.

---

3   Morgan Murrell, "Jodie Turner-Smith Had A Home Birth Due To 'Systemic Racism' In Hospitals, And It Proves Just How Scary Being A Black Woman In America Can Be," *Buzzfeed*, August 12, 2020. https://www.buzzfeed.com/morganmurrell/jodie-turner-smith-home-birth-decision

But it happens. A lot. And there are studies that show that my birthing experience is a lot like that of other African-American women who've had babies in hospitals."[4]

♥ ♡ ♥

PREGNANT AND SCARED

By: Monique

On the night of November 2nd, I was home alone, and hubby was at work. The dog and I were lounging on our off-white sectional couch in the living room watching television. By this time, I was thirteen weeks and two days pregnant, feeling much better since the nausea had eased and I had a cute baby bump to show. I went to use the bathroom and wiped: there was slight bleeding. I remember my hands trembling as fear struck me. I wiped again, just to make sure I wasn't "seeing things." I ran upstairs to change my underwear and put on a sanitary pad. I grabbed my toothbrush in case there'd be an overnight stay. Filled up Sebastian's water fountain, and I was out the door with keys and cellphone in hand. Luckily, we lived only twenty minutes from the nearest hospital. While on the way, I called hubby to tell him what happened, and since his business was close to the hospital, he arrived shortly after me.

I was not in any pain; I had yet to experience Braxton Hicks contractions, nor had I felt the "popcorn" movements of our growing baby. I texted my parents and my older sister to let them know what happened. After hubby arrived, I ex-

---

4   Denene Millner, "Birthing While Black: An Experience I'll Never Forget," *Huffington Post,* January 30, 2012. https://www.huffpost.com/entry/african-american-birth-story-hospital_b_1231247

plained to him what had transpired at home. As we sat there, both of us scared to death, I remember thinking to myself, *This cannot be the end; we did not come this far to lose this baby.* I repeated that phrase to myself until a nurse called me for vital checks. She asked if I had any pain today before the bleeding, and I told her no. She asked if I had been doing heavy lifting or anything, I said no again. I disclosed that I was a high-risk pregnancy because of my baby being conceived through IVF and that I was hypothyroid. The tech arrived and transported me to the ultrasound room to get images of the baby. They needed to make sure there was not an impending miscarriage. I felt myself getting anxious again as the tech prepped my belly. As soon as our baby's image appeared, I could see he/she kicking and moving around. My mind was put at ease, and I knew everything would be all right. Two days later, I went in for my appointment with the OB-GYN. She explained that sometimes women experience light spotting to medium bleeding during pregnancy. Her main concern was to check if the placenta was intact and make sure there wasn't any rupturing. According to the ultrasound, my placenta was close to the cervix, not previa, which is why I had experienced light bleeding.

My next appointment was at nineteen weeks with the radiology department to perform the anatomy scan. This visit would also reveal our growing baby's sex. The last time I saw our little pumpkin, he/she was still tiny, but now, our baby looked like a "real" fetus. The scan took about an hour and I was enjoying every moment! I could have stayed the entire day to watch my baby move, kick, squirm, and suck its thumb. I now had images to connect with the "popcorn" and "fish in water" movements I had been feeling since sixteen weeks. Before the tech goes underneath the baby's legs, she asked if we wanted to know the sex. Hubby and I turned to look at one another and he said, "It's up to you." I thought, *Ugh, great leaving it in my hands.* So, I told the tech, "Yes, I'd like to know." There it was, our baby's genitalia, clear as ever. The tech stated that the law did not allow her to disclose our baby's sex, so the radiologist called us from the waiting area and confirmed that we had ourselves a growing baby boy! Not only was this our first baby, but it was a boy! Hubby was proud and left with his head high to return to work while I stayed behind to receive the paperwork. I called my parents first and also sent text messages to my mom since she was still in school with her students.

My dad called and his words were, "Is that my granddaughter growing inside your womb?" I laughed and said, "No, Dad, you've got yourself a third grandson!" Dad was hoping for a second granddaughter. I called my sister at her desk and yelled, "VORA, IT'S A BOY!" She quietly whispered, "Yay!" and giggled. I said to her, "You know, after these years since our brother's passing, who would have known daddy would be blessed to gain three more sons through us." We began to ugly-cry over the phone. My niece called me later that day and said, "Am I still the favorite granddaughter?" I laughed and said, "Yes, Rae, after twenty years, you're still Pop-Pops only granddaughter!" She was happy.

On January 3rd, 2017, I saw my OB-GYN for the twenty-two-week check-up, and by this time, my belly button was protruding and I was looking like an expectant mother. My doctor performed an ultrasound. She asked how I had been feeling and stated I would visit her once a week during the third trimester. I was so freaking happy I decided I would treat myself to lunch. But, little did either of us know, it would be the last time we would see one another until after my baby was born.

It was Saturday, January 14th at around 10:30 pm. I was on the couch once again, hanging out with Sebastian, watching television. I got up to use the bathroom and what I thought was urine was blood, gushing. I felt no pain and no cramps. I jumped up to change underwear and put on a sanitary napkin. I gave Sebastian some water and food, while I called hubby to tell him I was making my way to the hospital and to meet me there! I grabbed nothing but my purse, keys, and cellphone. I was out of the door and called my sister. She was still awake; I told her, "Call daddy and my mother for me so I can drive!" I traveled as fast as I could and hoped there would be no red lights along the way. Finally, I arrived after what seemed like a one-hour ride. A nurse took my vitals immediately. I was not in any pain, and I would have to wait for a room. My phone was blowing up with calls from my parents and sister, asking if I had made it safely. Once I was in a room, the doctor came in, and she stated that I might be in premature labor. I was twenty-three weeks and six days. I was thinking, *There is no way I can have this baby now; he is still too young!* My mind was in a whirlwind and I could barely see straight enough to look this doctor in the eyes and listen. After a visual examination of my cervix, since it was too risky to check with her fingers, she said that I might be as much as three centimeters dilated. She asked for my insurance information, so I gave her my card. She went into another room to call and find out where the insurance company wanted me transferred, since they were not a level four hospital. I was given steroids for the baby's lungs, magnesium to stop premature labor, and penicillin. Hubby arrived just as I was being transported to the labor and delivery unit. Once there, the nurses attached me to monitors. Omar Jr. was kicking and jumping, letting me know he was okay. The sound of his heartbeat coming from the monitor gave me the peace I needed to close my eyes and sleep. By Sunday evening, baby boy and I were doing great. His measurements and vitals were on point and consistent. A high-risk obstetrician came in and did a second evaluation.

I was one centimeter dilated; Omar Jr. was footling breech (feet at the cervix, head above the navel), which I already knew and was common at his gestational age. My sac was not bulging but intact with plenty of fluid for him to dance around. I was to remain on bed rest at the hospital until the doctor was confident that my cervix would behave.

On Tuesday, January 17th, the nurses finally allowed me to bathe and freshen up; baby and I were doing just fine. The doctors were impressed with the strength of Jr's heart variations for a twenty-four-week fetus. I was hopeful but also human, rationalizing the things I could have done differently to prevent this. I began to feel as though my body was failing me, again! I wanted concise answers about why this happened to us, but no one had any to give.

Friday, January 20th, 2017 was Inauguration Day for the new President. I was feeling good, walking around my maternity room a little. I took a shower and shampooed my hair. Momma was looking scary after a week of being laid-up in the hospital. Once I finished my shower, I twisted my kinky-curly hair into a style to look more presentable. Hubby left and would return later that evening. I gave my Grandma Dee a buzz, and while on the phone, I felt a tightening in my belly that was very similar to Braxton Hicks contractions. I quickly finished my conversation with Grandma and went into the bathroom. As I was using the toilet, blood was dripping.

I had another tightening feeling in my belly. I wiped again—there was a lot of blood and I also felt a medium-sized bump hanging from my vagina's opening. I immediately knew it was my sac bulging, and this baby was coming whether I was ready or not! I jumped up from the toilet, waddled to the bedside phone, and paged the nurse's station. I yelled, "I think my baby is coming. The sac is bulging." My hands were shaking as I maneuvered myself back onto the hospital bed to wait for the nurse. Seconds later, two nurses rushed in, and I spoke faster than I ever have in my entire life.

I explained that I was using the restroom, and when I went to wipe, I felt my sac bulging. The nurse instructed me to lie on my back so they could check for themselves, and when the nurses looked, they could see that I was in active labor. The nurses immediately called upon the help of more nurses to transfer me to the labor and delivery unit while I was calling hubby to tell him what happened. With urgency, I said, "The baby is coming, you must get back here." It had been less than an hour since he left. He was at his place of business. I was shaking and trembling, but I managed to call my mother; I had no idea what she was in the middle of doing. I just yelled out, "Ma! The baby is coming. I am being prepped for surgery, I've already called Omar, and he is on his way back." She tried to ask more questions, but I could not focus, and I hung up on her. At this point, I was crying tears of fear and nervousness while I contacted my sister. Honestly, I do not remember if I texted or called her. So much was happening all at once. The staff told me it was time to go back to the OR for an emergency C-section—we couldn't wait any longer!

I was laying on the OR table thinking, *This cannot be the end; we did not come this far to lose this baby.* I sent a message to my baby: *Hang on, son; everything will be okay.* I awakened in the recovery room to the faces I love most—my husband, sister, mom, and dad. I remember my first words to them being, "Is he alive, did he survive?" The tears streamed down my cheeks and into my ears. I never knew this level of emotion. I do not remember everyone's reply; I recall them saying, "He will be okay, don't worry." The surgeon came in to tell us that the C-section went well and that my baby boy was in the NICU. I was relieved, thinking, *Okay, he must be alive.* I remember little of the conversation; we were in the post-op space since I was still coming down from the anesthesia. The next thing I can remember is hubby and my sister going to the NICU to see Jr. for the first time. I can only imagine what Omar Sr. must have felt—seeing his son for the first time, so delicate and fragile, and being unable to control what happens next. My heart truly ached for him. Upon their return to my post-op room, my sister came in and told me, "Mo, he is so little, and he has so much hair!" I do not remember hubby saying a lot. I think he was still in shock. He kept repeating, "I just left you, not even an hour ago." I never imagined after four years of infertility and then finally getting our big fat positive test result, that this would be our birth story. It often seems as if things are happening to test us.

The time finally came when I was allowed to visit the NICU for the first time. I was not allowed to walk yet, so I was wheeled there in the post-op bed. A receptionist behind glass doors and windows buzzed us in. We went past the receptionist's desk, stopped at the handwashing station, and then proceeded into the NICU behind two large doors. I saw clear incubators in well-organized pod areas, lots of monitors beeping at a medium level of sound, nurses on computers, and nurses tending to babies.

We arrived at my baby, who was covered in black hair that never got the chance to shed itself in utero. His skin was pink; I could see his tiny veins. The nurse explained the sensitivity of a micro preemie's delicate skin and immature nervous system. She stated that it feels painful for them to be stroked or rubbed. When touching him, I should rest my finger gently on his chest or allow him to hold my finger. She opened one door to his incubator, and I gently placed my forefinger from my right hand onto the center of his little chest. I felt my fingers move up and down as he breathed with the help of an oscillating machine. I said to him, "Hi, Omar, it's your mommy."

I cried. I cried for my man, my pregnancy, and most of all, my baby. I blamed myself because my body had failed him. It cheated him out of the opportunity to grow entirely within my womb, his safe place. One of his nurses explained the purpose of every cord attached to him and said that he was stable for now. I remember little about the rest of the night. My baby boy, Omar Farook Jr., was here. Arriving at 5:40 p.m., twenty-four weeks and four days old, he was one pound, nine ounces in weight and twelve inches long—my new hero.

♥ ♡ ♥

THE CULTURAL REVERENCE OF BEING MOMMY
By: Lola

A really, really huge piece of Asian culture is a concept called "sitting month," which means the month after you give birth, you are taken care of so that you can fully recover. There are two ways to go about it. First, if you are staying home, then your mother-in-law or your mom will cook for you, do your laundry—anything to help take care of the baby. You're freed up for a whole month. You get to relax and recover. You're not supposed to go out for a certain number of days and you're supposed to eat certain Chinese herbal medicines to refuel your strength and get your blood back. There are many traditional things that you do during the first month after giving birth and they're centered around your complete recovery. It's revered. It's expected. The whole culture and the whole society supports you and there are also little centers that you can go to if you don't have that support at home. At these professional centers, after you give birth, you pay them depending on how long you decide to stay. It may be a couple of days, but for some people, it's a whole month. You have a complete team to help you. Imagine having that kind of support. It's just incredible. In the United States, women are expected to go back to work after a couple of weeks . . . that's insane. In Canada, I feel like I've been very blessed as an immigrant and as a woman of color.

Imagine the positive outcomes if all women of color were given the support and care, during and after pregnancy, that they deserved.

The goal of trying not only to conceive a child, but to actually give birth, took a heavy toll on my mental well-being early on. I felt so much external pressure to physically give birth, as if biology was the only thing that could make me a mother. I remember the pregnancy that came after my second miscarriage, my OB-GYN told me that I would have to be on bed rest the entire time and that I would have to see a high-risk specialist every week to monitor my pregnancy. In this same conversation, she informed me that I would have to deliver via Cesarean section. I burst out crying. It wasn't fair. None of this was fair. I told her through my tears that I just wanted one thing in my pregnancy to be done the "natural" way. I wanted to give birth pushing my child into this world—I wanted what I felt was the true authentic birth experience. The doctor laughed, in a nice way. She put her arm around me and sagely said, "Candace, after nine months, you are not going to care how we get this baby out of you, and trust me, it's all authentic." As women, we are the creators of life. Do you remember that Jeff Goldblum line from the *Jurassic Park* movies? He says, "Life finds a way." Well, it's true. We don't have to physically give birth to a child to give birth to our families. We can find a way.

♥ ♡ ♥

THE BIRTH OF OUR FAMILY
By: Leia

As far back as I can remember, I always knew I wanted kids. I had a non-linear path to motherhood. When people think about motherhood, they think of a specific path, in a specific way. I wanted to have at least one child from my body; to see what features they would get from me, to see the mentality, the attitude to everything, all of that. I always wanted to adopt and foster children too. I know in a lot of relationships, both partners are not on the same page. One might say, "No, I can only have kids of my own," or, "I can only do this." It can be a struggle to get on the same page, but from the beginning, my husband said, "Yeah, it's great if we do have a baby, and if we don't, it doesn't matter. I choose you."

Being on the same page was very helpful. We tried for quite a few years to have a child. I got tested, he got tested, and the response was, "Oh, you guys should be able to have a baby, just relax, it will happen. Everything seems to work fine, there's nothing wrong with you." All the uncomfortable testing doesn't make you feel very maternal—it makes you feel poked and prodded, and it was a little demeaning. It felt so violating. It was the same for my husband, he wasn't feeling comfortable with the things that they're asking of him either. The only thing they told us was, "Oh, he has gentleman sperm." The sperm were very polite, as if to say, "No, no, after you." They weren't aggressive. I wasn't getting younger and was already being told I'd be having a geriatric pregnancy, which also didn't make me feel comfortable. The doctors said before trying IVF that we should do IUI, so I did one and I told the doctor I didn't want to do it anymore.

It was so uncomfortable and painful. It didn't feel like we were making a life together, that opportunity is technically still there, but I'm not rolling in money. To throw money out and then still have an outcome that may not be what I'm looking for wasn't worth the risk or discomfort for us.

We had money saved and could've dropped our savings on it or we could've gone into debt, but that's not how I wanted to become a mother. I got a lot of, "Oh yeah, you'll adopt and then you'll become pregnant." I kept thinking, *Why are you acting like it's the solution to not getting pregnant?* I wasn't going to adopt to "get" pregnant. It didn't sit well. So we came to the point where we pushed past the idea of me carrying our child. I mean, I'm forty . . . it felt like it was never going to happen.

It didn't feel like giving up, it felt like a relief. I was feeling like I failed every month when my period showed up. It was taking a toll on my well-being, my positive energy, on everything— it was just too much. We decided we were ready to move on.

We chose to start the process of becoming foster parents. With all the paperwork, it took years to get approved, but we finally got a foster kid in our home and I decided to focus on all the kids that spent time in my home.

Our second foster kid was only supposed to be with us temporarily; she was supposed to go back to her home. The parents were not in a position to be the parents she deserved. As foster parents, you need to have a big heart, because the goal is reunification. Our goal was always to give as much love as possible while they are with us. We knew being foster parents would be hard but worth it. This girl's parents just faded away. She's amazing, intelligent, and beautiful, I believe her parents realized that she was in such a healthy, happy, and thriving environment that they decided to back away. She is now on the path to be adopted by us. On a path to becoming our daughter. She's been with us over a year and a half, and she says it all the time, "I want to be here and this is my home." She calls us by our first names, which is what we introduce ourselves as, so it's what she knows. But yesterday was a big deal for me because she did some school work and she wrote Mom and Dad, which she's never done before. For me, it felt amazing. It was a big step.

REFLECTION

"When we address both the systematic disparities and implicit bias in both our society and our health care system, we can get to the point where being Black and pregnant is full of joy and free from fear of preventable death."

-Kamala Harris

In 2017, after having her daughter Alexis Olympia Ohanian via Cesarean section, Serena Williams nearly died from an undiagnosed, birth-related blood clot in her lung. Shortly after giving birth, she told the nurse she was in pain and gasping for air. Serena was extremely worried since she had a history of blood clots. The nurse wrote off her complaints as a bad reaction to the pain medication, which was making her confused. As an aside, I am still trying to figure out exactly how a person is "confused" about the pain they are experiencing. For hours, she pushed her doctors and nurses to perform a CT (computerized tomography) scan to check for clots. When the scan was finally administered it revealed that there was indeed a blood clot in her lung. It wasn't the scan that saved her life, it was the fact that she was able to strongly advocate for life.[1]

This was Serena Williams, Queen amongst Queens, and she had to fight to be heard.

Looking at how even relatively affluent Black women experience childbirth in New York City reveals a microcosm of a larger national problem: "A 2016 analysis of five years of data found that Black, college-educated mothers who gave birth in local hospitals were more likely to suf-

---

1   Maya Salem, "For Serena Williams, Childbirth Was a Harrowing Ordeal. She's Not Alone," New York Times, January 11, 2018.

fer severe complications of pregnancy or childbirth than white women who never graduated from high school."[2] Raegan McDonald-Mosley, the chief medical director for Planned Parenthood Federation of America, says, "It tells you that you can't educate your way out of this problem. You can't health care-access your way out of this problem. There's something inherently wrong with the system that's not valuing the lives of Black women equally to white women."[3]

Black maternal mortality rates didn't take a nosedive overnight and it's short sighted to blame it all on racism. A lot had to happen to fail Black women on such an epic scale. Aside from the implicit and explicit racial bias in the medical system, diseases like high blood pressure and diabetes disproportionately affect Black women. Socio-economic factors can also mean that prenatal care is either inadequate or non-existent. Finally, there is the underestimation and ignoring of Black women's pain. I had a radical hysterectomy in 2017 and was in the hospital for two-and-a-half days; they took everything—uterus, fallopian tubes, both ovaries, and even my cervix. I had a lateral abdominal incision since the surgeons were not able to operate laparoscopically. It was major surgery and it took me months to recover mentally and physically. You can't heal if your body is in pain and I was in pain. Every breath and every step hurt so much and took maximum effort. Still, I was sent home with a prescription for ibuprofen. My white husband, on the other hand, received a prescription for the narcotic painkiller Percocet after his outpatient laparoscopic shoulder surgery. I am not knocking his pain level; I'm sure his shoulder hurt. He took a full

---

2   Nina Martin and Renee Montagne, "Black Mothers Keep Dying After Giving Birth. Shalon Irving's Story Explains Why," NPR online, December 7, 2017. https://www.npr.org/2017/12/07/568948782/black-mothers-keep-dying-after-giving-birth-shalon-irvings-story-explains-why

3   Martin and Montagne, "Black Mothers Keep Dying..."

afternoon off work to nurse it back to health. I am just saying that after cutting me open, they could have given me a bit more than a few Advil.

When you are giving birth, the last thing on your mind should be whether or not you will receive the appropriate level of care due to the color of your skin. You certainly shouldn't have to entertain the thought that you or your baby may die in the process. Unfortunately, previously discussed racial basis and attitudes have left an ugly stain and enabled an incredibly toxic environment, making it scary to give birth while Black in America. A recent report shows that "almost one-third of Black mothers reported that they did not feel the delivery room staff encouraged them to make decisions about their birth progression. More than ten percent of Black mothers reported that they were treated unfairly during their hospital stay because of their race or ethnicity."[4] What I am trying to express is that it is not all in your head. Whatever feelings you are having are incredibly valid. The feeling that something is not quite right, or the lingering sense that you are being ignored or written off—that's very real. Our goal as women of color in the birth experience is to learn not to walk in fear but in power. All women deserve the best care possible when giving birth. We fall short as a society if we fail to acknowledge that we are failing Black women. As women of color, we know that we are more at risk, so let's take that knowledge and effectively advocate for ourselves and demand the care that we deserve.

Black mothers dying is not just an issue in the United States. The UK has a similar problem, which the campaign Fivexmore is trying to address. Fivexmore was founded by Black mothers Tinuke Awe and Clotilde Abe who also

---

4   Xenia Shih Bion, "Efforts to Reduce Black Maternal Mortality Complicated by COVID-19," *California Health Care Foundation* (blog), April 20,2020. https://www.chcf.org/blog/efforts-reduce-black-maternal-mortality-complicated-covid-19

created the hashtag #fiveMORE, which lays out five steps that women are encouraged to take:

1. Find an advocate or ally to support your claims
2. Get a second opinion on a diagnosis
3. Trust your gut feeling and do your research
4. Speak up about your concerns
5. Refuse to be silenced or ignored

The Fivexmore campaign believes that, "We must create an environment where women feel safe to raise their concerns without fear or judgment. Black women need to feel empowered and education is the key to this."[5]

Here in the United States organizations like the Black Mamas Matter Alliance work on a national level to advance Black maternal health justice. Created by a partnership between the Center for Reproductive Rights (CRR) and Sister Song Women of Color Reproductive Justice Collective (SisterSong), the Alliance is at the forefront of initiating a cultural shift through policy, advocacy, research, and advanced care for black mothers.

It can be easy to brush off the Serena Williams story as anecdotal. We all know the story of our friend's cousin's wife who had a bad birth experience. We may have read about the untimely deaths of Kyira "Kira" Dixson Johnson, Sha-Asia Washington, or Amber Rose Isaac because they got national press. We know in our hearts that anecdotes don't equal data. But the data exists, and the reality cannot be ignored. Not only are Black women dying in birth, they are dying unnecessarily. A Center for Disease Control (CDC) report from May 2019 on pregnancy-related deaths states that sixty percent of these maternal deaths were completely preventable.[6]

---

5 Habiba Katsha, "Giving Birth While Black: Why Is It So Much More Fraught With Danger?" Women's Health, July 21, 2020. https://www.womenshealthmag.com/uk/health/a33323338/black-maternal-care

6 "Pregnancy-related Deaths," Centers for Disease Control and Prevention, last reviewed May 7, 2019. www.cdc.gov/vitalsigns/maternal-deaths/index.html

None of this information should make you feel afraid if you are Black and pregnant. It should compel you to feel empowered to demand the care you deserve. "I don't want to sound an alarm that every Black woman who gets pregnant should be like, 'Oh, my God, I'm going to die.' Because that isn't the case," says Haywood L. Brown, M.D., President of the American College of Obstetricians and Gynecologists. "We just want people to know that 'I might be at a little higher risk because I'm a woman of color, regardless of what side of the track I'm on.'"[7] Never, ever doubt the strength of your voice, and never hesitate to use it for your own good.

Like many of you, I have my own story. I wasn't pregnant, but years earlier (before one of my IVF cycles) I had a myomectomy to remove several fibroids. They made an incision that looked a lot like a hysterectomy scar, except it was a bit longer. Post surgery, out of recovery and in my hospital room, I woke up feeling the effects of being cut wide open, but also feeling like something was really *off.* It wasn't just pain, it was the feeling that my body wasn't right. I told the nurse I was uncomfortable and she informed me that I should be fine and to try not to max out my morphine drip. When the anesthesiologist came by to do a post-op check on me, he didn't even enter my room or check my charts. He stood at the door, leaned his head into the room and asked how I was feeling. "Not well," I answered. "Yes, well, that's to be expected," was his reply as he walked away. Flash forward: what should have been a forty-eight-hour hospital stay turned into eight days of me suffering from a severe reaction brought on by complications with the anesthesia. I think back to that moment and wonder what more I could have done to demand that the anesthesiologist come into my room and listen to me.

---

7   Meaghan Winter, "A Matter Of Life & Death:Why Are Black Women In The U.S. More Likely To Die During Or After Childbirth?" *Essence*, October 2017.

But I was afraid—to cause a scene, to be a problem, to make demands, to be "that" woman that I was sure he had heard about.

The older, white woman in the room next to me actually had a sign on her door demanding that all doctors and nurses knock before they entered the room. She was in full hospital diva mode, demanding that hospital staff announce themselves and only enter with her permission, and the hospital staff were actually doing it. They were indulging her pettiness. Here I was, too timid to simply ask a doctor to enter my room or answer a question because I feared being given that dreaded label of "the angry Black woman." There is so much to unpack in my memory. The hospital needs to own its bias and make a huge cultural shift in treating patients. I need to own the loss of my own voice to fear. I allowed my health to be in jeopardy because I was too afraid to speak up. I was too afraid to speak up because I had spent a lifetime not being heard. That is the cycle we can find ourselves in as women of color. Serena Williams made a difference in her own health outcome for two main reasons: She had fully educated herself about her condition and she had a support system there to help her advocate for herself. Every healthcare professional I spoke with about this book said the exact same thing when I asked what was the best way that a woman could advocate for themself: educate yourself and find an advocate to help support you. Go in prepared and knowledgeable, have your records with you, and have someone there willing to support you and back you up. I learned at thirty-eight that the power was in me to make the outcome different. We have to be the ones to find our voices, speak up, learn to trust our gut, and to advocate for ourselves. As a Black mother, your life may depend on it; that's not hyperbolic, that is the truth.

Chapter Seven

INNER PEACE:
Finding Your Peace of Mind

*"Even as I hold you,
I am letting you go."*

-Alice Walker

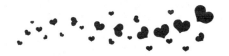

I am a deeply spiritual person. I don't align myself with any particular faith but believe in a Higher Power. I am optimistic but I don't believe in fairy tales, happily-ever-after, mystical or fantastic stories, and I certainly don't believe in miracles. I know that in real life, the princess most likely saves herself. After three miscarriages (six if you count all the occurrences of blighted ovum), nine attempts at IVF, one egg donor, and two surgeries to remove fibroids, I was in a place where I wanted peace and to say "screw it" to having a baby. I was done. Done with counting every day of the month, done with the pills, the shots, the patches, the tests, the transfers, the doctor appointments, the dreaded two-week wait . . . but most of all, I was done with hoping that it would all turn out well and I would be pregnant. My infertility was unexplained. I could get pregnant with IVF but I couldn't carry past the first trimester. It was starting to feel like every successful pregnancy test was merely a countdown until I miscarried. Infertility can crush hope. It crushed mine.

So there I was, bitter, angry, sad—so sad that it was palpable, like I was walking around wearing my sadness as a coat. There was a heaviness in every waking moment. The toll that loss could take on you mentally and physically was something that I had not been prepared for in trying to get pregnant.

I was, like so many of us, open to every suggestion to try to aid in my infertility journey. Drink "tea" that tastes like sludge from an abandoned garden—sure. Have the acupuncturist put electric charges on the needles to "shock" your system—sure. Follow a crazy diet—sure. Hang upside down by my ankles from the stairs while people slather me in yogurt—sure. My therapist suggested something out of the box; she told me about several clients she had referred to a medical empath. This woman was extremely sensitive to other people and their medical issues and she had received rave reviews. There was nothing I wasn't willing to try on my quest to do the impossible. I went in thinking it was going to be like those dogs you hear about that can sniff out cancer. I didn't think it would be an afternoon that would change my life.

I met with the empath, a lovely woman who, upon meeting me, gave me the warmest hug. She took my hands, looked me directly in the eye, and said, "I am so sorry for all your loss, I want you to know that you are the only one feeling this pain. All those souls felt so loved by you and they have moved on. Sometimes souls need just one moment and they are completely fulfilled."

I broke down crying, finally releasing how much had built up inside of me for what had been years at this point. The release of pain was jarring. A person can hold onto pain like a shield to block everything else out. My shield was down.

Over the course of the afternoon, she told me several things that she "sensed." There was a child coming to me, it just wouldn't come through my body. I was never going to give birth but I was definitely going to be a mother. A soul was waiting for me. This soul only wanted me for a mother but was stuck waiting because it couldn't come through my body.

I think about that afternoon often. I told my husband that night and he rolled his eyes and muttered something under his breath that sounded an awful lot like "that's bat shit crazy." In the retelling of this story, my husband now insists that what he muttered was "you sound crazy" (as if that is better). Trust me, I know how it sounds. It is silly, and strange, and a little bit kooky. In the end, the magic of that experience may have been as simple as hearing exactly what I needed or wanted to hear in that moment. What has stayed with me is the sense of peace and feeling of completion of a chapter in my life—that was what her words provided. She helped me let go and move on. I was the one who was stuck. Stuck in pain, stuck in one place, stuck in one singular idea of what motherhood would look like. I had to let go of the hope of ever carrying a child myself and it was hard to let that dream die. She gave me clarity and focus that I hadn't found anywhere else. She opened me up to the possibility that creating a family and being a mom did not have to look any specific way.

Getting pregnant was not the goal. What was important to me was becoming a mother and there is a whole world of ways to be a parent. Within months, miraculously, my husband and I welcomed our son through open adoption. Max was even born the week of what would have been the due date of my last transfer. He was my baby. The one soul that was stuck and waiting for me. The moment he was placed in my arms, I whispered, "I am sorry it took me so long, I've been waiting only for you, too." And in case you are wondering, yes, I do believe in miracles now.

Resolution is an extremely hard place to get to from where infertility can drop you off. If everything does not turn out the way you wanted or the way you dreamed, you may not feel as if the journey is complete. Resolution in infertility often means letting go of all the things that you have held on to tightly through most of your life. You won't find any peace of mind if you keep holding onto the pain in the past. You have to find a way, as difficult as it is to move through it; there is no shortcut to the other side of this process.

I have said it before and I will say it again, infertility is tough. It sucks and is unfair. It is somehow all out of your control. You can go through all the treatments, the tests, spend tens of thousands of dollars and still never get pregnant, never stay pregnant, and never have a baby. That's what's so incredibly scary, that loss of being in control and the knowledge that sometimes, no matter what you do or even how much you pray, it may not work out. You may find yourself grasping at any straw and putting your faith and belief into almost any hope that is offered. A mantra begins running over and over in your head like an incessant broken record: *Why not us? Why not me?* You want more than anything to be part of that elusive, successful group and to call yourself "mommy." Someone will always have something to say about the choices you make, and people will jump at the chance to give you advice. If you make your life about listening to them, you will definitely drown out your own voice.

IT'S A MARATHON, NOT A SPRINT . . .

By: Michelle

Think about running a marathon (even if you don't run, go with me on this one). Imagine how exhausting it would be to only focus on the last mile of the twenty-six mile race, rather than celebrating each mile marker on the way. The next mile seems a heck of a lot closer than the twenty-sixth one, doesn't it?

Marathons are as much a physical experience as they are an emotional one. Talk to anyone who has run a marathon and I'm sure they'll tell you that they needed to get their head on board just as much as their body. Infertility is exactly the same.

With infertility, you might not have the privilege of knowing how many miles, months, or years are going to be part of this journey, but you can choose to celebrate the mile marker right in front of you with each step. And it's equally important to get your head on straight, otherwise, you feel like you're in an endless spiral of feeling, like you're going insane all the time.

It may feel silly or crazy to celebrate milestones that may never come to be, but without doing so, it's hard to hold onto hope on this journey. This is the exact reason we chose to celebrate the little embryo we recently transferred; we had cupcakes and a small family gathering on Zoom. Whether or not it sticks around, it's here now and to me, that is worth celebrating.

♥ ♡ ♥

I FOUND MY PEACE

By: Alicia

One challenge God gave me in this journey was to decide whether I truly loved and trusted Him for who His word says He is, or did I just want a genie in the bottle. Did I simply fellowship with Him? Go to church and study the Bible for affirmation of who I was and to receive what I wanted? Honestly, at some point my faith turned from dependence and trust to, *Oh, can*

I have this, too? As my faith faltered, I began to reflect on what I had learned of God. And the Spirit brought certain passages and songs to my heart such as Jeremiah 29:9-14, Psalm 37:3-7a, and 2 Corinthians 12:9. I came to the firm decision that God was worthy of all praise. And so I began asking myself, what is Your purpose. And even though I did not receive a clear proclamation, I nonetheless began to believe my life had purpose in Him even if I could not understand it. Even if it was not the purpose I had envisioned for myself.

What could be more personal than finding exactly what brings you peace and comfort? This discovery is going to be different for everyone. One woman's peace is another woman's crazy. After my first miscarriage, I spent weeks wandering around in a haze of misery and sorrow. I spent a lifetime being informed that, as a woman of color, I had to stand up to adversity and pain in silent strength. I was the strong Black woman; I fully brought into the trope that was pushed upon me from birth. I knew that I had to be self-sacrificing and that my strength lay in being impervious to a lot of my feelings. Showing vulnerability meant showing weakness. I didn't have permission to be weak; I was the one being superwoman and holding it all together. Initially, I didn't even question doctors—I wasn't honest about my physical or mental pain. I was so entrenched in my inner dialog of being strong that I wasn't able to recognize the depth of my own depression. I don't remember how dark my depression got, but I do remember that my husband and my doctor were extremely worried about me. One night, over a dinner that I wasn't eating, my husband looked at me and told me that he couldn't remember the last time he saw me smile or heard me laugh. My doctor called a few days later and encouraged me to see a grief counselor.

Now, I have to take this time to say that if you are on this journey, I can't stress enough how important it is to have a solid support system. I did not "self-care" my way out. Having support saved me in every way. "Here's what I would want a woman of color suffering through mental anguish to know: You cannot inoculate yourself from your mental struggles by denying its existence. You must be proactive in finding support, even if that means going outside of your community of loved ones and seeking professional help. Going to a psychiatrist or therapist does not make you self-indulgent; it is a cognizant act of self-love and mercy for which you don't owe any explanations or apologies".[1]

It was my very first therapy session that gave me a path towards healing.

I had an evening appointment. It was an uncharacteristically cold and rainy Los Angeles night. I walked into the office and sat across from the therapist; with my head down, I told her the experience of my miscarriage, every horrible detail that was still seared in my mind. I spilled out all my pain and it felt like bile leaving my mouth. I was spitting out my complete misery with every word. I finished and sat there, staring at my shoes and waiting to hear all the familiar words I had heard before: that it was meant to be, that it was for the best, that we could try again. Things that had been said to give me comfort but did little to soothe the hole that had been ripped open in my heart. Instead, I heard a voice, clear as a bell: "Yeah, that sounds fucked up." *WHAT?* I looked up and locked eyes with the face belonging to the voice and she repeated,

1   Sara Ahmed, "As a Woman of Color, I Didn't Seek Help for Postpartum Depression," *Huffington Post,* updated July 31, 2020. https://www.huffpost.com/entry/postpartum-depression-women-of-color_n_5f22d76ac5b68fbfc87fe0be

"That sounds really fucked up, I am so sorry." Her words struck through me with the physical force of a gunshot. It was one of the most electrifying moments of my life. I stared right back and said, "Yes. Thank you, it was fucked up, it was completely fucked up." The dark cloud lifted. I took a deep breath, exhaled, and felt better than I had in weeks. Someone had given a voice to what had been stuck inside my head ever since I sat bleeding over a toilet in the early hours of that December morning, literally watching all that I hoped for, loved, and dreamed about disappear. It wasn't pretty, it wasn't what nice girls were supposed to say or think, but it was the truth—my truth—and it felt so good to acknowledge it for what it was: Fucked up.

Peace of mind came to me in a way that was completely unexpected, but was ultimately just what I needed to hear at a time when I was ready to receive it. I will say it again—one woman's peace is another woman's crazy. Find and live unapologetically in your peace.

REFLECTION

*"The truth is, unless you let go, unless
you forgive yourself, unless you forgive
the situation, unless you realize that
the situation is over, you cannot
move forward."*

-Steve Maraboli

Everyone has that one defining moment in their in-fertility journey. That sweet, serene moment no matter how brief, where the clouds part, the lens clears, and you see where you are. In 2017, I had my epiphany. You might say it was a moment of clarity. You could even say it was serendipitous. It came at a time when I was ready to hear what was being said. It was a moment when somehow, someway, it all just made sense. I call it the Gabby Effect. You haven't heard of this specific phenomenon before because I just made it up, so I will walk you through it.

By this point in time, other high-profile women of color had spoken up in power about their infertility bat-tles. Chrissy Teigan was tweeting about her infertility and the upcoming birth of her daughter. Renee Elise Golds-berry spoke about her infertility battle during her Tony acceptance speech. I had been fortunate to co-host a sup-port group with the sublime Tomiko Frasier Hines, a true pioneer, who was the first Black model to sign a major cosmetic contract and become the face of Maybelline. To-miko was one of the first women to speak out early and often about her powerful choice of egg donation to con-ceive her twins. As for me, I had spent years advocating and training others to speak on Capitol Hill about their infertility. At this point, I was already a mom and I was feeling so completely in control that I didn't think that anyone could tell me anything. Yet, somehow, through all of this, Gabrielle Union's voice broke through. I don't know why it was her voice and her story that hit me like a hammer hitting a gong, but it did. Maybe it was because we were roughly the same age. Maybe it was because I had loved her ever since she played Isis in Bring It On like a total boss. Maybe it was because she had always been honest in calling out her own bullshit and past toxic behaviors. I vividly remember a speech in 2013 where she spoke out passionately about how she had been guilty of breaking other women down if she felt that their success diminished her light. It is not easy to look deep into your own dark corners and adjust yourself and your behavior. She put in the work and I had always admired her strength in self-reflection. She felt authentic to me, especially when I was holding on so tightly to the illusion of the perfect life that I had created in my mind.

In 2017, my son was three; the adoption had been finalized for a few years. Max was a walking, talking, solid-food-eating, fully actualized kid. Tommaso and I were looking ahead to the crazy process of trying to get our kid into kindergarten in Los Angeles. We were thrilled to move past the toddler years. I thought I had this motherhood thing down. I know they don't give out awards, but seriously, I deserved some kind of plaque for surviving that first year when sleep was a distant memory and showers and make-up were almost nonexistent. I never aspired to be an Instagram-perfect mom, I was just trying to make it through the day most of the time. That first year almost broke me, but here I was making it through age three like a champ. I have lived through two rounds of toddler Hand, Foot, and Mouth disease and a pair of ear tubes. Life was (almost) beginning to feel like it had before we became parents. Tommaso and I had regular date nights and Max was potty-trained and more self-sufficient every day. My life was slowly becoming my own again.

All the pain and hurt of trying to be a mom was still there. Trauma doesn't just disappear. It lies deep in the background, bubbling below the surface—a small, annoying, dull headache that is so quiet and constant you almost forget it's there because it becomes a part of you and easy to ignore.

For me, it's the times when I think I have it all together that I am the most deluded. I wasn't fine at all. I was so immersed in living the fantasy of my perfect life that I had convinced myself I had moved on. After all, I was the one leading a support group and guiding other women through the experience. Of course, I told myself over and over, I had been successful in overcoming all my infertility obstacles. I was fine.

Here's the thing, moving on does not always mean that you have moved past the issue. I couldn't arrive at a place where I was healed unless I allowed myself to fully mourn what I had lost. Having Max, adopting my child, did not cure my infertility. My amazing son is a daily reminder to me of my infertility and my body's inability to function the way that it should. I had to face that fact to genuinely move on and be able to show up and be there for my family. I had to acknowledge how much I had lost and how much I still hurt. I had to stop kicking myself for feeling all the unresolved pain and guilt.

There was one pivotal early moment I recall very clearly: as a new mom of a four-week-old Max, I had audaciously shared in a Mommy & Me group how hard it was getting absolutely no sleep at night. Instead of the common ground camaraderie I was expecting, my new role as an adoptive mom was thrown in my face with a response that "I should just be happy that I was a mom and not complain about my baby."

Lesson learned, loud and clear. The only emotion I was allowed to feel since I was infertile, was happiness. Nothing else was going to be accepted or permitted. If

I didn't toe the line, I was going to be isolated in motherhood the same way I was isolated in infertility. I shut down. I slapped on a smile and lied to myself. The voice in my head told me that to move forward through every day, it would be better and easier to pretend that I was fine. That is what people wanted to hear and I was nothing, at that time, if not completely immersed in the false notion that it was my job to please everybody.

There are five stages of grief; denial, anger, bargaining, depression, and finally acceptance. While there are five stages, grief is not a linear path. There is no timeline and we all experience grief in deeply personal ways. For me, it was so much easier to deny pain than to face it, especially when people were demanding that I be strong. It came easy to me to deny pain after a lifetime of people downplaying my actual physical pain of endometriosis and fibroids. It was easier for my pain and hurt to manifest as anger when I did try to face them. I funneled my anger into my advocacy efforts. It became my brand. I told everyone who would listen that pure anger was my prime motivator. I used to make the joke in my speeches that anger channeled in the right way would lead to great results. It was a line that always got a laugh. Hiding my pain led to me constantly second-guessing every decision Tommaso and I made since I was diagnosed with infertility. For what it's worth, I am still second-guessing myself to this day. I have a list running through my head of all the choices or steps I would have taken if I could go back and do it all again. It is depression that took the biggest toll and has sat the heaviest on my heart through the years. There was a time during the constant agony of endless IVF cycles when just seeing a pregnant woman would trigger tears. I remember a particularly hurtful and hard day (I am now ashamed to admit) after a failed transfer when I wanted to physically slap every pregnant woman I saw on the street. One time on a trip to the grocery store, I saw a pregnant woman shopping with her biracial toddler and it was like looking into an enchanted mirror of what my life should have been. I left my cart full of all the pregnancy-inducing fresh fruits and vegetables in the produce aisle, ran out of the store to my car, and cried. I cried those hot, angry tears that come from deep inside with the gut-wrenching sobs that make it hard to catch your breath. That was a bad day.

My acceptance came three years after I had my child. It came while I was living in the dream of the life I had always wanted and fought so hard to achieve. It came in a clear defining moment of hearing Gabrielle Union talk openly and honestly about everything it took for her to become a mom. She was not the first woman of color to open up about infertility struggles, yet for some reason, it was her voice and raw emotion that cut through to me.

In the early 2000s, I had seen all the magazines and neatly produced TV packages about celebrity miracle babies. Often the most miraculous thing about them was how they lacked detailed information about exactly how the miracle had been achieved. Instead of comforting me, many of those stories added to the cacophony of voices making me feel far worse. It seemed to give ammunition and talking points to all those well-meaning voices trying to support me by telling me about all the women who got pregnant well into their forties and fifties: "Look at who just had a baby! See, you can do it too!" All the pictures and stories that focus solely on the end result, without the context of all the struggle, don't serve to move the needle forward.

Gabrielle Union's opening up sparked something in me. The effect her story had on my life felt personal. She put it all out there. The good, the bad, the ugly, the loss, the anger, the pain, and the frustration. She laid her life bare, without ego, shame, or reservation. Her story felt like a warm and understanding hug that I was able to collapse into. I know Michelle Obama had a very similar effect on a lot of women. So many women saw themselves in Michelle Obama's story that the instances of women seeking fertility treatment after her book came out rose almost 20% in some clinics.[1] That is the power of representation and that is what it means to women to see themselves in this experience.

Recently, my favorite comedian, Michelle Buteau was featured in a People Magazine story about her beautiful new twins. She spoke openly about her struggle to get pregnant and her experiences with surrogacy. I couldn't help thinking about how different that same article would have looked a decade earlier. There would have been the same glossy pictures but perhaps the article would have had flowery introductions to her beautiful twins and her smiling coyly while recounting her very special delivery. Luckily for all of us, today she proudly, boldly, and honestly recounted her experience with infertility, the racism she endured, and the path to surrogacy that resulted in the birth of her babies. She doesn't just mention the miracle, she walks us through it step-by-step, and openly discusses the fact that her road to motherhood was nothing like she had imagined.

Opening yourself up and being honest about where you are in your journey and your feelings will only help to bring good things to your life. The moment I told my infertility story on social media, it was like I was found. People from all areas of my life reached out to me to share their journey and losses. My take from hearing Gabrielle Union's journey was that you have to be willing to be open and vulnerable to find community and support. You have to be honest about where you are and your people will find you.

---

1   Katie Kindelan, "Michelle Obama effect' sees more black women seeking fertility treatment 1 year after 'Becoming,'" Good Morning America Website, December 17, 2019. https://www.goodmorningamerica.com/wellness/story/michelle-obama-effect-sees-black-women-seeking-fertility-67685029

My biggest regret is that I didn't open up and talk more about the pain and anguish I was going through during all my IVF cycles and miscarriages. Anger was the easiest emotion to connect to and process. I wish I had opened up about what hurt and let more people in during that crazy time. So many of us are going through the same things—my greatest wish is that we all begin to understand that we do not have to go through them alone. Remind yourself every day, the way Gabrielle reminded me, that you are not, and will never be, alone in your experience. When we speak up and support each other, we ultimately heal ourselves.

In the end, peace of mind came with peace within my body. Infertility took everything from me, even my uterus. After our four year battle to become parents, my periods returned with a vengeance. They were getting longer and more painful and I was still accustomed to suffering in silence and trying to make it through. What finally happened still haunts me to this day. One evening while Tommaso was out jogging and I was putting Max to bed, Tommaso returned home to find me passed out in a pool of blood on the floor of Max's bedroom with Max crying and saying "Mommy won't wake up." I had been having my period for twenty days and had collapsed. We don't know how long Max sat there with me, and I can't even imagine the fear he must have felt and tried to comprehend in his toddler mind. I went to the doctor the next day and the imaging tests confirmed the existence of several large fibroids. They had returned. This time my doctor's suggestion was a Radical Hysterectomy. That was the only way my doctor felt that the pain would stop. She wanted to remove everything: my uterus, fallopian tubes, both ovaries, cervix, and two inches of my vagina. It is a surgery usually reserved for cancer patients. She was afraid that if she left anything, the fibroids and endometriosis would just keep coming back. She wanted some peace for me. She did not want to keep operating on me for years. Her voice over the phone was soft, "You have lived your entire life in pain. I just want you to rest." I had the surgery and you know what? I woke up in my hospital room feeling better than I ever had after any previous surgery. They went through my existing myomectomy scar and because they took everything out, it felt like there was much less internal bleeding and swelling to recover from. It was a long recovery process and it took months to get back on my feet, but to be pain-free and period-free after a lifetime of suffering is worth every single hot flash that came my way. I may be minus a uterus, but living period and pain-free has been one of the most positively liberating experiences in my life. I lost a uterus, but I found peace.

Chapter Eight

RESOLVE:
Moving On, Finding Peace, Letting Go

*"There's a real strength and
ultimately liberation in knowing
when the time's right for you
to let it go."*

-Lauren

Threw one question that I get asked most is, "How did you know when to stop?" Infertility treatments can seem like a Ferris wheel from a horror movie. It can take you round and round, confusing you with incessant noise and delusion. The whole ride is going too fast to even think about getting off so you just hold on and it can be endless. Honestly, for me, I woke up one day and I knew in my heart I was done.

I was actually in the middle of a two-week wait, my reproductive endocrinologist (RE) had transferred three embryos this time. None of them were top quality and the hope was that at least one of them would stick. I had been through this nine times. I was so hyper-tuned to my body that I knew, I just knew, with every part of my being that it was an unsuccessful transfer. I was muddling through a two-week wait and it was so difficult. My age, plus the fact that I had lost so many previous pregnancies, made me so high risk that I had to spend my two-week wait on total bed rest. I was allowed to get up to go to the bathroom, but that was it until the blood test. I had already been informed by my obstetrician that I would be on bed rest for the entire nine months, culminating in a cesarean section. I wasn't angry or helpless. I wasn't even sad. I was just done. I was physically and emotionally exhausted. My body was weakened from surgeries and treatments. I had experienced a transformational time with the empathic therapist. I was ready to move on. It felt almost peaceful to be done. Of course, I did the thing that none of us are supposed to do during the two-week wait (but we all do it anyway): I peed on the stick. My husband was frustrated with me, telling me to wait until the blood test, that I couldn't know for sure, that each time I was pregnant I was getting closer and closer to the second trimester. It was the very first time in four years that we were not on the same page. He still had so much hope that he was not ready to let go of yet. We still had embryos and the RE was ready to interview surrogates and had forwarded us several profiles. Tommaso wasn't at the place where he was ready to give up. When you have put so much of your life into making an outcome happen, it can be so hard to let it all go. We had been fighting for years for our dream. For years, our only focus was getting pregnant. Everything else in our lives—friends, work, family, even each other—had become secondary. I don't think either of us even knew how to stop and let it all go, but at that point, I knew that I was done. Comedian Michelle Buteau said it best in her speech at the 2019 Glamour Woman of the Year Summit: "I didn't realize what I would go through emotionally. You know, it was just four years spending thousands and thousands of dollars. Countless shots. Bruised bodies, tired spear, a partridge in a pear tree. It was crazy. And after four years of doing that, I decided, okay. Having a handful of miscarriages and still trying to get onstage and find my happy is too hard for me. And I have to make this simple for myself. I have to find my joy. And so the only option I had left was surrogacy. And I'm not a control freak. But wow, you have never felt so out of control."[1] I remember calling Tommaso after I had gotten the blood test results and shouting into the phone, "I

---

1   "How Comedian Michelle Buteau Owned Her Decision to Use a Surrogate," Glamour, November 10, 2019. https://www.glamour.com/story/how-michelle-buteau-owned-her-decision-to-use-a-surrogate

told you I wasn't pregnant, can it just be over?" We both spent time isolated in our pain and tried to find closure in our own ways. When you have been of one mind for years through the same struggle with infertility and IVF, it is devastating to be in different places. We were both mourning the loss of what we thought our life would be like. We were the kind of people who had always made things happen in our lives and now we simply couldn't make a baby. We were mourning the loss of all our miscarried children—the kids that we loved so completely, even though we never had the chance to meet them. It took time, but we found our way back to one another. It was such a dark and lonely place to be without my partner. It was hard for both of us to be so far apart in our thoughts and our plans for the next steps, when ultimately we both wanted the exact same thing. We just didn't know how to get there. I think we both had to understand and come to terms in our own way with what we had actually lost.

By living IVF cycle to IVF cycle, how much of our lives did we miss out on along the way? "Okay," he said, "we're done, but we always talked about having a family. You don't need to be pregnant for that to happen. Let's move on together." This isn't a book about marriage, but I will share this piece of advice passed down from my father: Don't marry the person you can't live without, find the person you can live with. When we vowed "in sickness and in health," neither of us thought there would be so much sickness. My husband has been my biggest cheerleader and biggest source of strength throughout our lives together. He is the one who never let me give up. Through every surgery, he cherished my battered, broken body. He helped me dress, helped me walk, even helped me go to the bathroom, and would still tell me I was the most perfect person in the world. When I hated my body and my scars, he loved them perfectly. Every imperfect inch. When he had to hold me over the toilet and clean me up after I went to the bathroom, he still told me that I was the woman that he desired more than anyone else in the world. You can save the picture-perfect Instagram photos of couples staring deeply into one another's eyes and captioned with the words, "True Love." Give me a man that wipes your ass and still wants to have sex with you when you heal—that, my friends, is true love. Uncurated, imperfect, and certainly not the way we grew up imagining love to be, but it is for me. It's amazing, beautiful, and sustaining. We were already a family no matter how the story would end. We would spend the rest of our lives grieving what we had lost in our own ways, but we had found a new way to love and understand one another.

GRIEF IS NOT LINEAR

By: Dolly | Marriage and Family Therapist

Grief is not linear; it's not even a circle. It's like a big squiggly line—it's unpredictable and sadly it never ends. Of course, over time and with work, grief changes, it softens (not that it goes away). Grievers need to understand how someone died, and that's also true with miscarriage. A lot of women and men who have lost a pregnancy become doctors and scientists themselves, because they learn so much about the process, what needs to happen, the medications and injections. People can become unexpected experts after the miscarriage, with the need to understand what went wrong and what happened. Often people aren't allowed the space to process their grief. You can feel alone in it, not because you are actually alone, but because you are surrounded by people who don't let you talk about your grief. People can shut it down. People may say, "Oh, you're young. You can still have another," or "You can adopt." Whatever it is they say, the implication is that you should feel lucky. I tell people all the time to never say "At least you have this . . ." because it minimizes the importance of what was lost. People need to understand their grief and they need a place to be able to process it without others trying to fix it or make it all better. That's kind of the inclination for all of us—to try and fix it—and that's where therapy can be so great. I like to highlight the idea of group work, I think there's something super powerful to help people connect and to have a space to ask the scary questions.

We also get to certain ages and stages and our grief changes. Then we experience what some folks, like me, refer to as a grief tsunami. I'll give you my example: A year or two after my mom died, I was at the bakery and I saw the chocolate eclairs and I began to cry. They were my mom's favorite and I would often get them for her. It wasn't the anniversary of her death, there was nothing going on—there was just a tsunami of grief that hit me all of a sudden.

It happens out of nowhere. Something will hit and the grief will take you over unexpectedly.

The grief tsunami hits me in very surprising and non-obvious ways. The smell of rubbing alcohol will still trigger me. The first ten minutes of the Disney movie *Up* affects me so much I have to fast forward through it or leave the room if it is on. The first time someone in Target told me that Max looked just like me, it hurt me in a way

I didn't think was possible. I was so shocked that a comment so lovely hurt me so much. I was still carrying so much pain that a compliment shook me to my core.

Aside from the grief, there is also a rather large elephant in the room when talking about infertility or the resolution to my story. I sit in awareness of how much financial privilege played into every choice that was available to me in trying to have a child. Money and privilege can't be separated in infertility. Finances affect your diagnosis, treatment, type of clinic, and what choices are made available to you.

There is also an inherent racialized privilege to motherhood. If the narrative of infertility is affluent and white, the narrative to motherhood rides in the same lane. If you are white and have a large family, you can see yourself being celebrated, not only in your daily life but in representations held up for admiration in popular reality shows. If you are Black or Brown, you are more likely to be met with some negative stereotypes of your large family. I grew up in the 1980s where the term "Welfare Queen" had a distinctly racial tinge and was used to describe the Black matriarch of a large family.

THE HIERARCHIES OF MOTHERHOOD IN INFERTILITY

By: Nefertiti Austin | Author of *Motherhood So White: A Memoir of Race, Gender and Parenting in America*

The stereotype of Black women is that we are fertile from the day we are born until the day we die and that we have no issues getting pregnant and popping out babies whenever we want; that's a huge problem. That notion impacts everything:

the doctor's perspectives on Black women, as well as the attitudes of nurses and mental health professionals. Miscarrying is not my experience and I can't imagine the toll that it takes. For a woman to get pregnant and, for whatever reason, be unable to sustain the pregnancy must be traumatic. Then, if you want to talk to someone, a medical professional or therapist, about the loss, but you may feel that you can't, or feel uncomfortable with the idea, because you know they will not see you or your experience on the same level as a white woman's miscarriage. That has to be devastating. Many white doctors don't have the same level of empathy for Black mothers or Black prospective mothers because vulnerability and pain—physical or emotional—are reserved for white women. So, when you know that you will be confronting so much *stereotype* around the nature of your feelings, regardless of skin color, but especially because of skin color, it's very difficult to be forthcoming and to get the support and the help that you need. This hierarchy is incredibly problematic because it keeps us at the bottom. Another by-product of racial hierarchies within motherhood is that Black women aren't as open with one another about what they're going through. The shame is palpable and there can be a reluctance to share "Oh, I went to this doctor and she was terrible, but this person was warm, compassionate, and empathetic," or "I got the best advice from these people." This is the information that we need to share with one another. We have to remember that every woman's body is different, and talk about pregnancy struggles, because I think we associate all of that with white people and that's kind of what we're told; white women have those problems, not us. I think Black women might be harder on ourselves if we do have trouble conceiving because we've also bought into the myth that "I should be able to do this." At the risk of alienating white mothers, and making them uncomfortable, we need to talk about Black women's infertility and why this health issue is important to all mothers.

Tommaso and I were lucky that our privilege enabled a lot of our choices. His job came with insurance that covered infertility treatment up to ten thousand dollars. We thought we were going to skate by on that. Looking back at how hopefully naive we were, I can't help but laugh out loud. That ten thousand dollars was gone long before we even got to our first transfer attempt. It went like sand through open fingers. In total, we spent close to one hundred thousand dollars over four years trying to get me pregnant. We are not people who casually had that kind of money on hand to spend, but we were able to do nine IVF transfers and were looking at surrogates for our last three embryos. When we were through with IVF, we were able to move to private adoption. That is financial privilege. So is the fact that we had the choice to continue with treatment when something failed. For many women, treatment may stop abruptly simply because they can't afford to continue. There is very little solace in the cold hard facts. Even with all the money in the world, even in the best of circumstances, even if all the stars align, there is no guarantee that you will become pregnant, carry a child to term, and give birth. Welcome to infertility, where your money may make it easier, but that still will not make it happen.

Sooner or later, we all get to the place and time where we let go of the dream we've held on to so tightly. For me, I had to learn the subtle difference between giving up and letting go. Over and over in my head, my internal soundtrack was playing the words, broken, damaged, unfit, unfair. None of these words are true but if you say anything enough, the thoughts begin to find a home in your head. I am guilty of allowing that to happen. I think so many of us are told to never give up. I was told to never give up—that if I wanted something badly enough, I could never stop fighting for it. We are told to keep trying and eventually, through hard work, science, faith, prayer, blind luck, or divine intervention, if we never give up, we will get what we want. But, in life, that is not always true. I tried for years and was never able to carry a pregnancy past the first trimester. I also know more than one lucky lady that got pregnant on their first IUI or IVF. Sometimes things work out and sometimes they don't and as much as we want to, we just can't wish our dreams into existence. So the question remains, how do we let go without giving up?

♥ ♡ ♥

FINDING GRACE

By: Belinda

My husband and I have been together for twenty-four years and married fourteen of those. We also have a big family house even though it's just the two of us. I'm such an organized person; I plan for everything. I'd say that infertility has completely taken over. It changed my life—it's a different way of life and now I think, *Oh gosh, is this it? Am I ever going to be normal again?* It took a while, a couple of years, for me to realize that I could control how I felt. I could be grateful for what I had and, even though it hurt every day, there was still so much to be grateful for, and that I was still very blessed. That is what changed my mindset. I wish I'd learned that lesson earlier. My mom died in the midst of all of this. I think she's the only person apart from my husband who understood what I was going through. She could empathize because she wanted a grandchild more than anything.

I am Nigerian and in our culture, when you have your child your mom comes to stay. She will stay with you for at least a few weeks, if not a month. When we renovated our house, we had created the room for my mom to come and stay. I have been pregnant four times and lost every pregnancy. The third time I was pregnant, she came to stay. In a way, she was testing out the room, and it felt so nice to have her there. We never thought she would get sick and pass away. I am full of emotion—thinking about how I don't have any children and I don't have my mom. So Mother's Day is a nightmare every year. You feel every day that it's going to happen, there's hope . . . there is hope.

I AM STILL PERFECT EXACTLY AS I AM

By: Danielle | Life Coach, Reiki Master,
Divine Radiant Living

Let's put them together, side by side: Giving up and letting go. The energy within each term is very different. When you're giving up, a part of you feels like you're surrendering to something, but there's this negative energy behind it. There is this sadness, there is this grief, there is, in a way, a forced acceptance. It is a surrender that is not coming from your power, not from your heart saying this is what I think is best for me. You've been knocked down, you've been dragged, you have been beaten up, so you're giving up because you can't take it anymore. The idea of giving up has a lot of pain and suffering behind it.

When you are in a place where you can let go, you get to work through all those feelings. You can process in a healthy way how you're feeling disempowered and out of control with everything. You get to empower yourself by saying I see all that, I feel all that, I honor it, and I know that's not the journey; that's not a path I'm going to continue on.

Letting go is allowing yourself to willfully and consciously accept and surrender to the path unfolding in front of you. This path looks different, is completely unknown, may seem scary, and might be filled with fear, doubt, concern, and worry. Understand that you have choices for how to travel this path; say to yourself, *I have no control over this, but I'm still going to trust and have faith.*

There is a more positive, connected, even spiritual connection to letting go. There is a respect and an honoring to it, which is different from the feeling of giving up. If you imagine it, giving up looks like a person who's been dragged through the mud, who's gone through immense pain and suffering and can't go on any longer.

When someone has experienced loss over and over and over again, they must process the pain and suffering behind that, and if they don't get through to the healing stage, then it can feel the same as giving up. It's coming to a place of saying to yourself, *I have no choice in all this; there's nothing I can do*, rather than, *I understand this is the situation, and I'm going to move forward with a different option or alternative. I'm going to find peace and resolution in it.* Giving up doesn't have a peaceful resolution—it feels more like a comma instead of a period.

When you let go, there's a period. You understand that the story has ended in this way and it opens you up to a new story in a completely different way than what you imagined. If you think you are giving up, you will not have a clear path to finding a peaceful resolution because you haven't worked through your grief to find peace.

Sometimes we get stuck in our grief because we want a sense of control. I think we want to have control over our bodies, and we want to have control over our stories. There is this delicate balance between what we actually have control over versus what we don't. There is also a worthiness and a perfectionist aspect, and that comes from some level of unresolved trauma in infertility. As women, we may have felt we had to be able to have children or that there's a defect in us if we can't. So now we feel imperfect if we can't create a child naturally. As an Hispanic woman, coming from a cultural background where fertility is customary, as soon as you're married, the question is when are you having the baby. If you're not able to meet that expectation, the sense that there's something wrong with you—that you have failed your family, failed yourself, failed your husband—is real and painful. Culturally, it starts to call into question everything about your existence and it becomes a very existential process. Not a lot of people want to question their identity; it's a challenge. Healing is not easy. It forces you to look in and question, *What is my truth?* In some ways, it's a lot easier to give up, curse the world, place blame, or use different coping strategies instead of doing the inner work—letting go and saying, "This is what it is."

To get to the point of letting go, we have to reassess our identity, reassess our definition of what's perfect, what's normal, and what's acceptable, not just socially but also within ourselves We have to be able to look in the mirror and say, *I am still perfect exactly as I am, I'm still worthy and deserving of becoming a mother, if that's the route I really want to take. I accept that my path to motherhood may look different and that my life may not include having children of my own.*

If you wanted to be a mother, how do you honor that without having children of your own? Maybe it's taking care of nieces, nephews, and baby cousins—being there for them, supporting family members, giving yourself the opportunity to help, and them the opportunity to rest. For those of us who continued with the motherhood journey, however, we know that having support and community is huge. Maybe for you, community means volunteering as a big sister or big brother. Maybe it means becoming a foster parent. Maybe it means going into the hospital as a volunteer for the babies who are born with health issues or born addicted and they need someone to hold them. It's allowing yourself the creativity to explore what your life looks like, and knowing that you don't have to birth a child to be a mother. Mothering is about nurturing and nourishing; it's about caring and that starts with how we care for ourselves and how we can take those properties and qualities and share them within our community. Whether that's with friends, family members, hospitals, different organizations—that choice is yours. But before you can achieve this, the first step requires taking a deep look inside.

Find a way to connect with others. I think it helps to connect with other people and hear their stories to know that you're not alone. To discover where this journey ends, you have to do the inner work, and preferably with someone else alongside you, guiding you, whether it's therapists, your religious or spiritual mentor, a grief counselor, support group, or a trained pregnancy loss professional. No one else can give you validation or acceptance, it has to come from yourself, and then from there, you decide to write the rest of your narrative, in a way that honors you.

IT'S A FIGHT FOR YOURSELF
By: Keisha

Be your own advocate! It's a fight for yourself, you know your body better than the doctors . . . When something's wrong, something's wrong. Don't just take their word for it. Pray all the way through everything. Just fight. Fight for yourself. I feel like, especially with my PCOS (Polycystic ovary syndrome) diagnosis, I just accepted it and I didn't ask many questions. I still don't quite understand exactly how they came to the diagnosis because I don't have any of the other symptoms.

Fight, do your research, and ask a thousand questions. When they become annoyed, ask more questions. That would be my best advice.

I FOUND MY VOICE
By: Halima

How do I advocate for myself or how do I become a better advocate? The first thing I had to do and to acknowledge was that I was a woman of color in a white supremacist healthcare system. Acknowledge that, be aware of that, and be aware that it will inevitably influence your experience navigating the system. You have to be aware of that because the thing is, if you're not, you're going to think, *Maybe I'm not in pain, maybe that person who said that I have to go see a doctor was just exaggerating, maybe I'm overthinking.* You're always going to think that way if you don't have an awareness that being a woman of color is going to inevitably influence your experience. Once you are aware of that, then you can be on guard, then you can protect yourself.

♥ ♡ ♥

FIVE EFFECTIVE WAYS TO ADVOCATE FOR YOURSELF

By: Dr. Theresa Buckson, OB-GYN

I believe that there are five ways to advocate strongly for yourself as a patient:

1. Verbalize that you think something is wrong. Especially if you are over thirty-five, don't wait, don't lose time. Speak up and tell your doctor that you think something is wrong. Do not be afraid to have an honest discussion about your fertility issues.

2. Find a doctor, find a clinic that will listen compassionately to you and address your needs. If you feel that you're not being served, don't be afraid to change doctors or clinics.

3. Educate yourself. Find out what is going on with your body and how underlying health issues (fibroids, PCOS, endometriosis, etc.) can affect your fertility. Take care of those issues.

4. Understand and have a solid financial plan. There is a large financial burden to all of this.

5. Have your partner get tested as early as possible. Although women have to do the heavy lifting in infertility cycles, almost half of infertility cases are due to male factor infertility.

If it seems unfair that so much of this falls on the shoulders of us as patients and as women, that's because it is. It is unfair. It is just another part of infertility that totally sucks. The road through all of this is not easy. It is messy work, it's uncomfortable to talk about, and no one is guaranteed a happy ending. That is exactly why we have to talk about it. We have to create the space where we normalize these conversations. We have to acknowledge all the experiences unique to women of color to take away the shame and stigma. All of that helps in learning, as a patient, when it is time to push forward and recognizing when it is time to take a breath and let go. Don't allow nice-sounding platitudes from others to guide you through this journey. You have a voice and never doubt it's supreme and distinctive power. Show up, speak out, claim your place, and do not let anyone hijack your message. I can't say this enough, advocating for yourself and others is what will make a difference in fertility access, treatment, and outcomes. No matter what color we are, we share the hope of becoming mothers. That is what binds us together. The voices in this book may be centered around women of color, but the stories are universal.

Toni Morrison famously said, "If there's a book that you want to read, but it hasn't been written yet, then you must write it." You get to write your own story of your journey and your struggle. You will know when it's right for you to stop and move on if you are listening to your voice. And sometimes . . . you just need to stop, so you can push reset.

REFLECTION

"Some days are just hide under your blanket and try not to lose your mind days. And that's okay. And that's enough. And that's strong too. And you can be resilient some other time. And whoever says otherwise can KYA. People so often ignore the arm strength required to wave the white flag."

-Regina Townsend

It is little things that have helped me move on. I found special ways to remember and honor all of the babies that I never had the chance to hold in my arms. I keep an empty silver frame on top of the bookcase in Max's room among all of the other family photographs. It is next to the picture of me and Max's birth mom—me smiling with both hands resting gently on her growing belly. I always tell Max that was the moment we met. I say that I put my hands on her stomach and called out to him, "Max, it's Mommy, I can't wait to meet you," and that he kicked his legs so I could feel them to say, "Mommy, I will see you soon." It has become his origin story and I like to remind him that most superheroes are adopted too.

I also have a thing about marshmallow fluff. I don't like marshmallows in particular, but every time I was pregnant, I would have symptoms really early on. I was very nauseous and tired, and I reveled in every symptom. Nausea was proof that I was pregnant. Nausea was great! I also started craving marshmallow fluff, of all of the weird things to crave. So, Tommaso would buy it—it comes in this six-ounce little plastic jar. I would eat it from the jar with a spoon in one sitting without any shame or embarrassment. The baby loved marshmallows and I had to give the baby what they wanted, right? I paid attention to everything I ate, but marshmallow fluff was my sweet indulgence. I had saved the last jar of marshmallow fluff that Tommaso had bought for me during my last pregnancy. I kept it for years in the kitchen cupboard and every time I'd open the kitchen cupboard I'd see it, and I'd smile because that was a tangible reminder of the pregnancies. Even after having Max, looking at this jar was a reminder that I HAD been pregnant and, for some reason, that was a comforting thought. If you're infertile, having that possibility is huge.

One Thanksgiving, I opened up the pantry and I saw the jar sitting on the shelf. I was making a sweet potato soufflé from a recipe handed down from my grandmother. I grew up in California, but my people were from Georgia so all my Thanksgiving recipes were things I saw on the table at Grandmommy's house. There were collard greens, black-eyed peas, cream corn, ambrosia, biscuits, fruit cobbler, and marshmallow-topped sweet potato soufflé. So that Thanksgiving, I found myself reaching for the jar of fluff and wanting to spread it on top of the sweet potato soufflé. I have to interject that the shelf life of fluff is ridiculous—it could probably survive a nuclear blast. The fluff was still in fresh fluff condition.

So, I opened up the fluff and I gave some to Max on a spoon (with only the small nagging thought that I was giving him basically a spoon of pure sugar) and it felt really symbolic to me. I spread it on top of the souffle and watched it melt down in the oven. I had let go of that hope of being pregnant. I had my son. We were done; we were a family of three. I had to completely let go of all of it. It's hard to accept that your body doesn't work the way you want it to, and I think people who haven't experienced infertility don't understand the pain of that reality.

Every time I look at my son, it's also a reminder that my body wasn't able to do what it was supposed to do to bring him here, but I'm so lucky to have him and I'm so lucky I got to experience all of those moments his birth mother allowed me to have. Seeing him being born was the most amazing thing I've ever experienced in my life, but it also hammered home that my body wasn't capable of that.

It's weird now to open up the kitchen cupboard and not see that specific jar of marshmallow fluff staring back at me. I continue to do the marshmallow fluff every year at Thanksgiving. Also, every now and then, I still eat it from the jar with a spoon.

Chapter Nine

BEING AN ALLY:
Providing Love and Support Without Being a Jerk

"If it sucked for me, I can't even imagine how hard infertility must be if you're not white."

-Woke White Friend

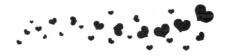

In centering the experiences of women of color, voices that have been kept below the surface get the elevation they have long deserved. I began this book by pointing out that as infertile women, we all share a common pain. For women of color, the struggles may look different and the reality feels different, but we are all ultimately trying to reach the same goal. I am grateful for the allies I have met along the way. Nothing matches the infinite power of women reaching out to help other women. I am sustained and comforted by the stories of my Black and Brown sisters and I am grateful for the women that stand beside us in this struggle.

♥ ♡ ♥

HOW TO BE AN ALLY

By: Sarah

As a white woman, I know that my experience with infertility is different. I'm aware of many (although likely not all) of the ways my outward appearance gives me privilege and I constantly struggle with knowing how to respond or what to do about it. I have done my best to be a good friend to the women in my life; there is a unique bond amongst those of us who have struggled to create the family we desire. We know all too well the often-unspoken heartache, shame, rage, self-doubt, and isolation that comes from being unable to conceive or bear a child of our own. In that, we are equals. And yet, women of color are even further isolated in their experience because of systemic racism, stereotyping, and bias that exists in ourselves and all areas of our society, including the healthcare system.

So, how to be an ally to a woman of color who is struggling with infertility?

Believe her. Believe her when she tells you the doctor is dismissive of her or treats her differently. Believe her when she raises concerns about her health or her body. Believe her when she knows something just "isn't right." Honor her intuition and acknowledge her experience. Believe her. Listen. Offer support—which isn't the same thing as offering solutions—and make sure that support is free from spiritual bypassing and "whataboutism."

Honor the ways your experiences are the same as women: women who want children; women who want children and are struggling with infertility; women who want children and are struggling with infertility in a culture where people are often unaware or insensitive to the challenges women face when trying to have a baby. In that, you have a shared experience that unites you.

Understand, acknowledge, and accept the ways that your experiences are different. Being a woman who struggles with infertility is already isolating. Being a woman of color struggling with infertility is compounded by a multitude of issues that I, as a white woman, will never experience or fully understand. I have a responsibility to know that and to do my part to dismantle the systems of racism within myself, my family, my community, and in the myriad of institutions that perpetuate the false narratives on which racism is built.

Believe her. Honor what unites you. Be a good friend. Listen. Learn. Do the work.

♥ ♡ ♥

THE SWEET SURRENDER TO FREEDOM

By: Jessica

My journey was filled with heartbreak and ambivalence. On repeat. My husband and I terminated two very wanted pregnancies. We hesitated. We had our living son. We hesitated. We wanted to give him a sibling. I miscarried twice in the two years we tried, without the help of science. We hesitated again. As a privileged white woman, it was not lost on me that our trajectory would look different had we lived in a different state, different city, if we had a different socio-economic background, or different skin color.

I thought about crying Uncle. I may have even said it out loud. I considered being done with trash cans filled with pregnancy tests, done with hoping for two lines, done with the look on my OB's face when he isn't able to find a heartbeat on the Doppler.

But instead, I dug deep. Like Bill Murray's titular character Bob in the film *What about Bob?*, I told my problems that I was on vacation. I took six weeks—not six weeks of hesitation, but rather six weeks of freedom. A freedom and identity outside of this existence between living life, creating life, and death. A literal mid-life crisis. I gave no thought as to how my day-to-day might impact pregnancy. I used nail polish with chemicals. I drank wine. I drank caffeine. I worked out a lot. I saw a crystal healer. I got facials that might not have been safe for a pregnant woman. I bought legal weed. I got a tattoo.

When my six weeks were over, I was refreshed. I was ready for one final attempt with IVF. One round only. I was prepared for the possibility that this path may end in life, may end in death, or may just end.

Ambivalence. Excitement. Fear. Grief. Relief. The narratives that go along with these feelings all existed simultaneously, yet there was no through-line. All separate stories happening at once. I discovered I could accept these feelings as different aspects of a whole experience; I was not in control. For the first time in years, I felt truly free. I surrendered.

Uncle.

♥ ♡ ♥

FINDING A SPACE WHERE YOU FEEL COMFORTABLE

By: Kristin | Fertility Nurse, Fertility Massage Therapist, Fertility Doula, Fertility Patient

One of the most important things to consider when seeking fertility treatment is finding a fertility practice where you are extremely comfortable with your doctor and their staff. Finding the right clinic for you is going to be one of the biggest measures of your success. This is an environment where you may be spending a lot of time during your fertility journey. It is important to surround yourself with people you trust, people who support you in every way, and most importantly, people who ensure your voice is heard. In preparation for your upcoming appointment with your chosen fertility practice, make sure you gather a complete history of your fertility medical records and beyond. Certainly, your specific fertility history is most important, but a thorough medical history about you, in general, is also very important. There may be some information included in your general medical history that may seem insignificant as far as infertility goes, but it may in fact be a small key that opens up a big door when investigating why you are experiencing infertility issues. This does not just include a thorough medical history for the female half of this equation, but also a complete medical history for the male half. You are both in this game of making a baby and both of your medical histories are equally important. Being able to openly discuss your medical history can be a huge help. If you have had a history of fibroids or endometriosis since a young age, these are very important factors to discuss with your fertility professional.

A prudent fertility doctor will want to review these medical records prior to your consultation. If you end up in a consultation with a fertility doctor who has not taken the time to review your personal records before your arrival, then that doctor is not the person you want to be responsible for your fertility treatment. This should raise a huge red flag that this practice is one to avoid. You want a fertility doctor who wants to get to know you from the initial meeting. It is not only important for the fertility professional to know the details of your medical history, but it is equally important that this doctor gets to know you. What are your hopes and dreams for starting your family? What things are important to you as you navigate this intimate and important journey? Your fertility treatments should be tailored to you and you specifically. There is no room in fertility for the cookie-cutter mentality. Learning all about you will give them an informed place to start, which is very important when considering the financial aspect of your treatment. If there have already been low-level diagnostics or tests performed that need not be repeated, or treatment that was not fruitful in the past, you may not want to go through the expense of repeating it if it is truly unnecessary. You do not want your treatment to look like that of every other person who is coming through their door. In my many years of being a fertility nurse, I have yet to see even one fertility plan that was the same as another. Every single fertility journey is different.

I would also make sure that that doctor is well-educated on the medical factors that are issues on a more regular basis with African-American women and men.

One thing to address before you even step foot into a fertility practice is this: are you and your partner both on the same page? Are you both willing to discuss subjects that can be difficult to talk about with others? Oftentimes, men have the worst problem because of their pride.

Infertility for men is often a silent struggle. It is very hard for men to find any true support amongst their friends or family members when going through fertility treatment. They are mortified to find that they potentially do not have "super swimmers," saying things like, "I am not telling any of my brothers that!" This also holds true for women of color experiencing infertility. Culturally, it is believed that women of color face a stereotype of being more fertile than other women. This assumption brings a stigma to infertile women. Women of color often find it hard to find their own support from friends and family when everyone around them is getting pregnant and starting their family with ease. Women of color do not often see themselves represented in this world of infertility. They do not hear their friends and family members talking about it. It is not sensationalized when a celebrity woman of color has sought infertility treatments.

Women of color even struggle to find other women of color practicing as reproductive endocrinologists. How do you find common ground when your friend, your sister, or your cousin become pregnant while in the same room with their partner? That common ground is even harder to find when other women of color are not talking about their own infertility journeys with their cohorts because it's a taboo subject. Studies have shown that women of color are disproportionately affected by infertility in terms of prevalence, utilization of treatment, and access to care.

Another reason women of color are hesitant about seeking fertility treatment is because of practical concerns. Fertility treatments are extremely expensive with no guarantee of success in the end. Insurance companies are becoming better in their coverage of infertility diagnoses, but they are certainly not perfect, and there are always out-of-pocket expenses that need to be considered. In addition to the uncertainty of insurance coverage, there is the time lost from work for multiple office appointments and procedures that accompany this path of infertility. This also contributes to the financial worry that surrounds fertility treatments.

Lastly, I would like to address a term that I coined while navigating the infertility whirlwind; it is called the "Fertility Tornado."

My inspiration for the Fertility Tornado came from my time as a fertility nurse and a fertility patient. Whether you are a nurse or a patient, when you are in the throes of anything fertility-related, it feels like you are in a tornado. As a fertility nurse, there is so much to organize for each patient each day. Appointments, procedures, schedules, medications, labs, forms, insurance, etc, etc, etc! The list goes on, and on, and on. As a patient, you deal with a very similar list that encompasses every breath you take. It affects your health, your marriage, your intimacy, your mental status, your finances, your schedule, your family life, your friendships, etc, etc, etc! The list goes on, and on, and on. There is not one corner of your life this infertility thing does not infiltrate. Trying to keep everything straight is like being in a fertility tornado. I am certain that I am not alone in feeling the way I do about this world of fertility. Make sure that you always remember why you are here: To start or grow your family, not to beat the problem.

Infertility is one of the most difficult issues a couple or anyone looking to start or grow their family can face. It is extremely important that you walk this journey with your eyes wide open. Establish a united front for how you will navigate this together. Working together as a team is imperative. Always be there for each other and never play the blame game. Each of you needs to share the burdens and the joys. Be in tune with your partner so you can build them up when the road is rough—and it will be.

Lastly, be kind to yourself and, most importantly, each other. Remember that the reason you started down this road is that you want to start or grow your family with the person you love most in the world. Do not lose sight of that.

My biggest ally remains my husband. He really is my partner in crime. I am lucky that I have a relationship where I like my partner as well as love him. I hope that you have the same kind of love and support in your life as well, whether from a friend, spouse, or partner. I imagine that it would be devastating to have to go through any of this alone.

When I had my hysterectomy, it was a lot to process. It felt like I was losing everything that biologically made me female. I didn't know how to feel—happy, sad, resigned, cheated? I mostly felt lost. It was Tommaso who yet again was able to make sense of the senseless and said, "None of that made you a woman. You are a woman simply because that is who you are—in your head, in your heart, in your soul. There is nothing that they can take from you that could make you any less of a woman. Your biology has nothing to do with the fact that you will always be Candi." With these words, my husband, my best friend, proved once again that the nineteen dollars I spent on my Match.com membership was the best financial decision I ever made in my life.

Full disclosure: being thrown into instant menopause at forty-seven was not pretty. My body changed overnight. I have a permanent pooch that no amount of Spanx can hide. I live in an extra thirty-five pounds that no amount of exercise can make disappear. I have more acne now than I did as a teenager and, before I finally threw them out for not sparking joy, I used to stare at my old jeans and remember when I could fit them over my thighs. So, I would be lying if I said that I didn't sometimes miss the person that I used to be, but this is where I am now. It's not the life I ever imagined, but it's the life that I am living and learning to love.

So yes, infertility sucks. It kicked my ass. It knocked me down but it didn't take me out. I am still standing here. Ready for the fight. We've got this.

REFLECTION

"Unless you have been through it, there isn't much you can say to someone with infertility issues. It's better to just give loving support instead of explanations, suggestions, and reasons."

-Dana Russell Reimann

You can hope, you can pray, you can have all your finances together, and you can do everything right, yet still, it may not work out the way you want it to. The most frustrating thing for me was, it seemed that becoming pregnant and having a baby came down to blind luck, and not being lucky hurts. A lot. And I get it, I know it can be confusing to be an ally. The desire to help but not knowing the right thing to say or do, and badly wanting to show you care, but it feels like you are putting your foot in your mouth every time you try to be supportive.

So, maybe the answer is actually simple—just show up, be present and don't try to *fix* anything. You can let your infertile friends know you care by simply asking them what they need and not assuming that you could possibly know what is best. I understand that you think you may have some great suggestions but trust me, we have thought of it (probably have tried it), and we really don't need your advice—we just need support. When I say support, I mean for you to truly support their decisions even if they are not the decisions that you personally would make.

I certainly don't speak for every infertile man or woman, but I can tell you what would have been, and what was not, helpful for me. I wish more people had shown up to support my husband, my partner—a man who experienced every loss that I experienced yet had no one check in on him. Also remember that infertility is NOT a female specific disease. Twenty to thirty percent[1] of infertility is male factor infertility. Show up and support the men who may suffer in the silence that toxic masculinity (related to fertility and virility) can produce. Resist the need to try and make someone feel better by minimizing their pain and trauma. Allow them all the time and space they need to process their hurt without forcing them to cheer up. Try not to link their infertility to some divine plan of whether or not they are meant to be parents. It is not helpful to tell infertile couples to "just adopt"—I am an adoptive parent—I powerfully chose adoption as a way to build my family; Adopting my son was *not* the consolation prize for being infertile. Finally, if you take nothing else away with you from everything you have read in this book, please hear this—NEVER, under any circumstances tell an infertile person to "Just Relax!"

I am extremely encouraged and supported by how the extraordinary community of women (and especially women of color) have really forced a seat at the table to show up and shoutout on this subject. For far too long, infertile women have been living in a cloud of disenfranchised grief—that is the grief and loss that is not acknowledged by society; We are not supposed to talk about miscarriage, so we suffer our losses in silence and isolation; We are not supposed to talk about infertility so we think that we are completely alone.

There is a very specific link between what you see, what you read, and what you begin to believe. Today, I do see some people that look like me, telling my stories, understanding my pain, helping to heal my loss. I also see women who don't look like me genuinely coming to the

1   Ashok Agarwal, Aditi Mulgund, Alaa Hamada,Michelle Renee Chyatte, "A unique view of Male Infertility around the Globe." *Reproductive Biology and Endocrinology,* April 25, 2015 https://www.ncbi.nlm.nih.gov/pmc/articles/PMC4424520/

table and beginning to listen. It is not everything, but it's a solid start. We are all forced into membership of a club that we never wanted to be a part of, we all deserve to have our stories heard. Change has to begin somewhere and after all that I have been through, I find myself at a place where I am hopeful and at peace.

Epilogue

One Last Thing...

"Perhaps the path to healing begins
with the three simple words:
Are you OK?

-Meghan, The Duchess of Sussex

It can be hard to open up after a lifetime of being told not to air your private business in a public space. I have learned that one voice can speak to the experience of many. I am full of gratitude and humbled by the bravery, strength, and vulnerability of the women who have shared some of the most private and painful experiences of their lives within these pages. For everyone who spent time on Zoom video calls with me, or took time to write down their story, sharing the pain as well as the triumph, I am incredibly grateful. As I said in the very beginning, I don't just want to tell my story, I want to share yours.

I am grateful for the allies who contributed their stories, support, and guidance. Women who fully acknowledge their privilege in navigating the path to motherhood, but know that for it to get better, they have to be willing to stand and advocate for all women. Also, for the partners who have been steadfast in their love and support—people who stand beside us and shoulder our pain and loss.

I recognize that I stand on the shoulders of giants. The amazing women who have come before me to speak out about race and infertility moved the conversation forward to create a space for a book like this to exist. I always acknowledge that there is no single, monolithic experience for minority women going through infertility, but there is a common thread that allows us to show up for and support one another with a particular understanding.

I am grateful for the women who declined to participate. I understand, acknowledge you, and respect your choice. Cultural issues, secrecy, and shame are still very much in play in the larger public conversations about infertility. You may feel alone but always remember that you are standing alongside other women who know exactly how you feel. I hope that the stories and experiences shared here have helped you to feel strong, heard, seen, and validated. In some small way, I hope that this can be part of a beginning—a small impetus toward removing the shame from the discourse. For real and effective change to happen, we have to be willing to sit in a place of discomfort and start the conversation. I share the story of my journey to motherhood as often as I can, and as loudly as I can, because I never want anyone, for even one moment, to feel like they are alone.

So, let's begin. I'm passing the microphone. Start where you think your story begins. Infertility is . . .

Allow yourself to fill in the blanks.

RESOURCES AND SUPPORT

Think of this list as a starting point. It is far from complete but a great place to begin when looking for resources and support. Use it as a key to open up larger doors.

RESOLVE
The National Infertility Association   *Resolve.org*
RESOLVE exists as a space to learn and educate yourself, find support, donate, or help take legislative actions to support the infertility community.

FINANCIAL SUPPORT AND GRANTS

The AGC Scholarships   *agcscholarships.org*
AGC is a nonprofit group committed to providing both advocacy and scholarships for those struggling with infertility in the United States.

Angels of Hope   *angelsofhopeinc.org*
Creating Miracles Infertility Grants provide monetary assistance to help close the financial gap that stands between married couples and the fertility assistance required to conceive a child.
Everlasting Imprints Child Loss Grants provide headstone and burial cost assistance to area needy families who suffer the death of a child from stillborn to the age of three.

Baby Quest & Baby Quest Kenya Moore's Gift of Life Grant   *Babyquestfoundation.org*
This foundation offers financial help to diverse groups undergoing fertility treatment. *Kenya Moore's Gift of Life Grant is open to those in the Detroit area.

The Cade Foundation   *Cadefoundation.org*

Since 2005, the Cade Foundation has provided information, support, and financial assistance to help needy families overcome infertility. Their grants can help families with the costs of treatment and adoption.

Chicago Coalition for
Family Building   *Coalitionforfamilybuilding.org*

The Coalition for Family Building offers Family Building Grants to eligible individuals and couples to help defray the financial challenges of infertility treatment, adoption, or third party reproduction.

Must reside in Illinois, Indiana, Iowa, Missouri, or Wisconsin.

Fertility for Colored Girls   *Fertilityforcoloredgirls.org*

This organization offers three grant options to help build the family of your dreams:

- FFCG Gift of Hope
- FFCG Kindbody Grant
- Baby Launch Grant

Journey to Parenthood   *Journeytoparenthood.org*

This group helps couples and individuals dealing with infertility achieve their dreams of becoming parents by providing financial and emotional support along their journey, as well as providing education and resources.

They strongly believe that all couples and individuals who wish to love and care for a child should not be stripped of their dream or limited due to financial constraints. Journey to Parenthood's dream is for those struggling with infertility to realize their dreams of parenthood. What comes so naturally for many should not be such a hardship for millions of others.

Pay it Forward
Fertility Foundation   *Payitforwardfertility.org*
Applicants are selected that are uninsured for fertility treatments. The grant amounts vary among the grant recipients, and partial and full grants can be awarded.

FINANCED INFERTILITY TREATMENT PROGRAMS AND DISCOUNT RX

The ARC® Affordable Payment Plan™   *Arcfertility.com*
The ARC® Affordable Payment Plan™ helps with fertility financing and the cost of IVF or IUI. This program helps make infertility treatment more affordable through an extended payment program. This option allows you to make manageable monthly payments.

EMD Serono Fertility Lifelines
Medication Program   *Fertilitysavings.com*
The Compassionate Care Program provides eligible patients savings based on income. Eligible patients may save 25%, 50%, or 75% off the self-pay price for the following EMD Serono products:

- Gonal-f ® (follitropin alfa for injection) 10% off per 75 IU
- Ovidrel ® PreFilled Syringe (choriogonadotropin alfa injection) 10% off per 250 mcg
- Cetrotide ® (cetrorelix acetate for injection) 10% off per 0.25 mg

Fertility Finance   *Fertilityfinance.net*
This organization provides friendly, affordable, stress-free, financial solutions for fertility treatment. Fertility Finance specializes in providing patient financing services for all fertility treatment options. Their easy, convenient loan process and competitive rates ensure the financial as-

pects of treatment are not an obstacle to achieving your dream of a family. Fertility Finance offers a wide variety of loan options, allowing you to attain the necessary financing required to make your treatment affordable.

SUPPORT GROUPS AND BLOGS

The Broken Brown Egg   *Thebrokenbrownegg.org*
The Broken Brown Egg Inc. (NFP) is an awareness and service organization founded in the summer of 2009 to increase awareness of African American Infertility and Reproductive Health.

Divine Radiant Living   *Divineradiantliving.com*
This multifaceted organization is focused on healing. Divine Radiant Living provides services from specialists like intuitive spiritual advisor, medical intuitive medium, and reiki master. Here's what they have to say about their services:

> *However you found yourself here, thank you for being here and for taking this next step. I believe in G-dincidences and in the alignment of energies and of making desires a reality when we are ready for real and permanent change to occur. A part of your spirit led you here, even if the Why is not yet clear to you. Listen to what speaks to you, listen to your inner intelligence, listen to that feeling inside of you that no longer wants to keep with the status quo. Together we can help you feel free from what's been blocking you; uproot the pain, suffering, or trauma of your past; and offer you tools and resources to navigate your healing journey—all by helping you heal yourself on a deeper, more soulful level. You are the Healer of your Life.*

EM-POWER Donation   *Empowerdonation.com*

This group is an ***education*** company dedicated to increasing awareness, empowering choice, and fostering understanding for everyone involved in embryo donation.

Fertility for Colored Girls   *Fertilityforcoloredgirls.org*

This group provides education, awareness, support, and encouragement to African American women/couples and other women of color experiencing infertility and seeking to build the families of their dreams. Additionally, FFCG seeks to empower African American women to take charge of their fertility and reproductive health. Chapters in several states provide monthly private support group meetings, participate in National Webinars, and advocate for women/couples struggling with infertility in their area and abroad while connecting to the larger FFCG Movement.

Monica Bivas, IVF Coach   *Monicabivas.com*

Monica will help you walk your IVF journey by being the missing link between you and your clinic. Free 30 minute Discovery call and free resources.

My Brown Baby   *Mybrownbaby.com*

My Brown Baby is irreverent, funny, and full of posts that make you think—maybe even make you say, "Amen."—it reminds you of what's going on behind your closed door, with your family. It's a place where African American parents, parents of black children, and their opinions matter and are heard, respected, and revered. For their poignancy and strength. For their intelligence and authenticity.

Parents Via Egg Donation   *Pved.org*

PVED was created and designed for the parent or the parent-to-be by other parents and parents-to-be. Whether you're just starting out on your journey to parenthood, are already pregnant, or are now a parent, this is the right place for you.

thrIVF   *Thrivethroughivf.com*

Here's what Michelle has to say about what thrIVF has to offer:

> *I'm Michelle, an IVF support coach and your biggest infertility journey cheerleader. You can basically think of me as your built-in IVF journey bestie. I'm here to help you calm the negative spiral and find the strength to hold out hope for your miracle. I know it feels like infertility robbed you of all the things that once brought you joy—that it turned your life upside down. This road will be hard—there's no way around that. But infertility doesn't have to control your life. I'm here to show you that it's possible to get off the emotional roller coaster, leave the overwhelm behind, and get your life back. Together we can find a little more joy in this journey and peace in your heart.*

Your Trusted Squad   *Yourtrustedsquad.com*

Your Trusted Squad is a curated resource of the most trusted health information, apps, gadgets, and online healthcare services available to help you if you are planning to get pregnant in the future or are currently trying to get pregnant.

PODCASTS

Black Girls Guide to Fertility
blackgirlsguidetofertility.com/webisode

Black Women and Infertility
stitcher.com/show/black-women-and-infertility

Black Girls Guide to Fertility
podcasts.apple.com/us/podcast/black-girls-guide-to-fertility

Infertility and Me
infertilityandmepodcast.com

Sisters in Loss
sistersinloss.com

FACEBOOK GROUPS AND PAGES

Black Fertility.................................*@BlackFertility*

Black Women & Infertility...*@blackwomenandinfertility*

The Broken Brown Egg..............*@TheBrokenBrownEgg*

Fertility for Colored Girls....@FertilityForColoredGirls

Filling Empty Wombs "FEW".....@fillingemptywombs

Fruitful Fertility..............................@fruitfulfertility

Sisters in Loss.....................................@sistersinloss

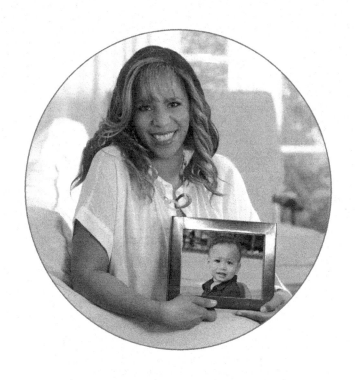

Candace Clark Trinchieri

ig: @infertilitystories
www. infertilitystory.com

After four and a half years, nine IVFs, two surgeries, countless miscarriages, a failed attempt at surrogacy, and one egg donor; Candace Clark Trinchieri and her husband are the parents of a son through adoption.

For over a decade, she has worked tirelessly to advocate for infertility access and affordability. She has served as an Ambassador for RESOLVE, The National Infertility Association, as well as National Vice-Chair Policy and Education for RESOLVE Advocacy Day. She has spoken passionately before members of Congress and Senate on behalf of infertility treatment and access for men, women, Military families, and the continued passage of the Adoption Tax Credit.

Home in Los Angeles, Candace co-founded Infertility Warriors with Tomiko Fraser Hines; this monthly support group was open to all women with a particular focus geared to the concerns of women of color.

With her husband and son, she is one of four stories featured in the documentary film One More Shot about her infertility and journey to motherhood.

Check out Mama's Gotta Grow!
Co-authored by Candace Clark Trinchieri

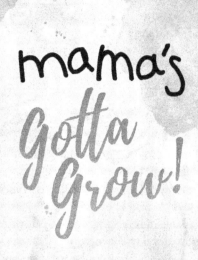

Available Fall 2021
www.goldenbrickroad.pub

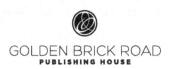

GOLDEN BRICK ROAD
PUBLISHING HOUSE

Link arms with us as we pave new paths to a better and more expansive world.

Golden Brick Road Publishing House (GBRPH) is a small, independently initiated boutique press created to provide social-innovation entrepreneurs, experts, and leaders a space in which they can develop their writing skills and content to reach existing audiences as well as new readers.

Serving an ambitious catalogue of books by individual authors, GBRPH also boasts a unique co-author program that capitalizes on the concept of "many hands make light work." GBRPH works with our authors as partners. Thanks to the value, originality, and fresh ideas we provide our readers, GBRPH books have won ten awards and are now available in bookstores across North America.

We aim to develop content that effects positive social change while empowering and educating our members to help them strengthen themselves and the services they provide to their clients.

Iconoclastic, ambitious, and set to enable social innovation, GBRPH is helping our writers/partners make cultural change one book at a time.

Inquire today at www.goldenbrickroad.pub

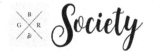